BRACES
DONE
RIGHT

T0272769

DR. PAUL R. WHITE

BRACES DONE RIGHT

THE FIRST TIME!

What Every Parent **MUST KNOW**
When Choosing an Orthodontist

Published by Advantage, Charleston, South Carolina.
Member of Advantage Media Group.

ADVANTAGE is a registered trademark, and the Advantage colophon is a trademark of Advantage Media Group, Inc.

Printed in the United States of America.

10 9 8 7 6 5 4 3 2 1

ISBN: 978-1-59932-935-2
LCCN: 2017964419

Cover design by Melanie Cloth.
Layout design by Megan Elger.

This publication is designed to provide accurate and authoritative information in regard to the subject matter covered. It is sold with the understanding that the publisher is not engaged in rendering legal, accounting, or other professional services. If legal advice or other expert assistance is required, the services of a competent professional person should be sought.

 Advantage Media Group is proud to be a part of the Tree Neutral® program. Tree Neutral offsets the number of trees consumed in the production and printing of this book by taking proactive steps such as planting trees in direct proportion to the number of trees used to print books. To learn more about Tree Neutral, please visit **www.treeneutral.com**.

Advantage Media Group is a publisher of business, self-improvement, and professional development books. We help entrepreneurs, business leaders, and professionals share their Stories, Passion, and Knowledge to help others Learn & Grow. Do you have a manuscript or book idea that you would like us to consider for publishing? Please visit **advantagefamily.com** or call **1.866.775.1696**.

To Drs. Ron Roth, Bob Williams, Larry Andrews, Ron Roncone, David Sarver, and Bill Arnette for your tireless dedication to the profession of orthodontics and for sharing your vast knowledge with an orthodontist who wanted only the best for his patients. You will never know the impact you've had on my career and on the lives of the thousands of patients who have benefitted from your teachings.

And to my beautiful wife, Allison, who put up with me being away from home so much in my pursuit of a "better way."

TABLE OF CONTENTS

Foreword

From the Founder of Excellence in Orthodontics

My name is Dr. Dustin Burleson. I'm an orthodontist and the founder of Excellence in Orthodontics. My reasons for becoming an orthodontist and forming a national organization for exceptionally successful orthodontists leading the field in both clinical and patient care—instead of becoming a veterinarian or handsome movie actor or professor of poetry—are easily found at ExcellenceinOrthodontics.org, if you're curious. They might matter to you.

But this book is about *you*, the parent, and your son or daughter, not about me. It's about information you need to know to make intelligent, responsible decisions about your child's health, appearance, self-esteem, and social interactions … of a permanent, lifelong nature. Does your child really *need* braces? If so, when? If so, who should you trust to provide his orthodontic care? How will you know you're not being ripped off?

This book isn't *Fifty Shades of Gray*. It just can't be that exciting. But if you take the time to read this book, you'll know how to confidently and correctly make whatever decisions you need to make about your child's orthodontic care.

It's *not* 1982.

To start, we're no longer dealing with heavy, ugly, tight, painful metal braces—every visit to have them tightened was another round of torture; they were hard to put on, hard to keep on, painful to remove, and it was irritating having a list of foods and activities to avoid for a long period of time. If your child needs braces now, the experience won't be anything like it was when you were a kid. He won't even try hiding under the bed and have to be dragged kicking and screaming to the car to visit my office.

Not only has *everything* about braces changed, but now all braces are created differently. So try to get that horrible, metal-mouth image out of your head. You're probably aware of invisible braces, maybe by a brand name: Invisalign. That's what prompts a lot of patients to call or email me in the first place. However, Invisalign is but one of a number of options to be considered to get to *the* best, customized, and personalized answer to your child's needs. You don't want to equate this to buying something over the counter: "Hey, give me Invisalign. How much?" It's more complicated than that. But it's a good representation of modern braces. They can be (nearly) invisible, pliable and with lighter steel, safer, and even self-removable for hygiene or sports and easily put back in place. They're not painful and achieve more certain results in a shorter period of time.

When I was growing up, a lot of kids didn't get braces they really needed and their parents let them off the hook, either because they believed their child couldn't tolerate the pain or because the cost was just beyond the family's budget. Now that braces are virtually painless, what about the cost?

Today's far better braces cost *less* than the one-size-damn-well-will-fit-all, metal-mouth braces of the '60s, '70s, and '80s. They cost as little as one Starbucks drink a day for a year, rarely more than twice that, and there are a number of different payment plans available if needed. So, that second hurdle is a lot lower than it was when our parents encountered it.

In other words, the first of my two introductory messages is: *relax.*

I've got your back. It's going to be okay—better than okay, easier than okay, and more convenient than okay. Orthodontic procedures *won't* hurt your child, and he or she will surprise you by not complaining it does. It's *not* going to hurt your bank account; you won't be reduced to a backyard stay-cation next summer and the summer after that. It's *not* going to be a maddening maelstrom of appointments of uncertain length, or hours in a waiting room: no emergencies from broken wires and loose braces, no time out of school, and no time away from work. Not at *my* office.

More Than Just Braces

My second introductory message is: this is about more than just braces.

Orthodontic care for a child, preteen, or teen is more than just correcting crooked, crowded teeth with braces. That's like thinking diabetes only needs attention when feet have to be amputated, or getting tires checked might be a good idea after being stranded with a flat at night while it's pouring rain.

"We appreciate all your efforts in helping Penelope achieve her beautiful smile. Our experience has been very enjoyable. Everyone is very friendly and we truly appreciate your flexibility given our busy schedules. We loved the fact that Dr. White made us wait until the right time for our daughter to start her treatment. That gave us confirmation that she was going to be in good hands."

-J. CASTANOS

Orthodontic checkups *by an orthodontist*[1], starting at age seven or eight, are a proper part of child rearing. In many cases, prevention is less troublesome and less costly. Even if you're late getting your son or daughter in, it's still possible they won't need braces and that other treatment options will do. But if they do need braces, the sooner you know of the options, the better.

This is also about more than just braces because it impacts psychological and emotional health, not just oral health. This is discussed later in the book.

Why It's Important

1. Straight teeth function better, are easier to clean, and are more likely to last a lifetime.

2. People with straight, well-aligned teeth can avoid gum disease, which has very serious health ramifications.

3. Properly aligned jaws reduce the risk of temporomandibular joint disorders (TMJ), which can ruin sleep or cause chronic headaches or migraines.

4. Both kids and adults with great smiles feel better about themselves, and that can greatly increase their confidence.

Some parents put off orthodontic treatment, but these irregularities and problems do *not* heal themselves. *This isn't acne; they don't grow out of it.* The problems only grow worse and harder to resolve with age.

---

1   All orthodontists are dentists, but dentists are *not* the same as or suitable substitutes for orthodontists. Read on to find out more.

Don't Ask Them to Hide Their Smile

Never smiling isn't easy in an age of selfies and social media. Children can become self-conscious—painfully self-conscious—and embarrassed. "No thanks, Mom, I'd rather just stay home."

Teen suicide has skyrocketed since social media shaming and bullying rose to ugly prominence. Teen depression affects everything from getting the good grades needed to get into a good college to first dates, first loves, and enjoying (or hating) their childhood and teen years. But it doesn't stop there. Uncorrected, bad smiles go with them to college and into their career.

This isn't just cosmetic either. It's also medical and can be a serious detriment to their health.

So, read on. Be informed. Be able to ask smart questions and do the right thing. I guarantee you'll be much better able to correctly and confidently make good choices for your family through this book.

Dr. Dustin S. Burleson, DDS

Founder, Excellence in Orthodontics

Clinical Professor, The University of Missouri Kansas City School of Dentistry, Department of Graduate Orthodontics & Dentofacial Orthopedics

Adjunct Professor, The Children's Mercy Hospital, Kansas City, Missouri, Department of Cleft & Craniofacial Orthodontics

Director, The Rheam Foundation for Cleft & Craniofacial Orthodontics

"The staff at White Orthodontics is phenomenal! They care about each patient and treat you like a friend. We were so impressed with their professionalism and quality of care. We could have gone to 'cheaper' orthodontists but we wanted it done 'right' the first time."

- J. FORD

Introduction

BOB'S TWO DAUGHTERS are patients of mine, but I hadn't really looked closely at Bob's own teeth until he made an appointment for himself. He told me, "I knew you knew what you were talking about when my daughters got started with treatment. Everything you said made sense. But it wasn't until I read your book and started thinking about my situation that light bulbs went off."

Bob explained he'd had braces as a teenager; his doctor had removed four of his permanent teeth to reduce crowding rather than expanding the jaws. But his smile is narrow, in contrast with the big, beautiful smiles we gave his girls. Even worse, he'd lost two more teeth because of the pressure that his bite put on them, and now he was having gum problems. He'd lost bone around all of his teeth because of the pressure, and his dentist had told him he was going to need another extraction. Bob's not slack about his oral hygiene; he visits his dentist every three months and flosses daily—yet in spite of his best efforts, his mouth is falling apart, because proper balance in his bite was never established.

1

"The crazy thing is, when I got my braces off, my teeth were straight," he said, "Now look at them." Not only are his teeth crowded, they're extremely worn down. Unfortunately, I had to tell him I couldn't help him; there just wasn't enough bone remaining around his teeth to allow us to move them.

I wish I could tell you that Bob's case was unusual, but it's not. For instance, a woman in her thirties came to me recently. She'd gone to another practice because she had TMJ (temporomandibular joint) problems. They had put braces on her teeth and made them straight, but they never got her bite right, and she was still in pain. So, just two months after getting braces off, she'd come to us for relief. We did TMJ therapy first to get her muscles to relax, and she's currently feeling better, but now her teeth don't even come close to fitting together, and she will need surgery to correct her bite.

It's not only adults who have these issues. A girl we treated had a sister—a junior in high school—who saw how much better her sister's teeth looked than hers, and complained to me that though she'd only been out of braces for a year, her teeth were already getting crooked. Now she wanted to do braces again, and this time, she wanted them done right. We showed her "before and after" pictures of many patients, because the difference is so striking between the smile she had after her first set of braces and the smile she has now. She told me, "What's funny to me is your 'before' pictures for my teeth were another orthodontist's 'after' pictures!"

Why do some people get better results than others?

Many people assume that all orthodontists are alike, but that's just not true. Orthodontics is a lot like cooking: two chefs might start out with the same sack of groceries, but one cooks a gourmet meal while the other's dish gets tossed in the trash. Why? Talent and training are critical elements; doing braces right the first time requires an artist's eye, a willingness to go the extra mile to diagnose correctly, and to treat what you find properly. In our practice, we use a lot of instruments and tools that most orthodontists don't. It's not the standard of orthodontics—it's well above the standard. The tools we use are similar to the ones a well-trained restorative dentist would use if he was going to put crowns on all of your teeth, because he'd also be changing the biting surface of every tooth. Not every orthodontist is as careful as we are about making sure your bite works as it should—even though the initial results they get might look good, they won't wear well—and that's where troubles can start.

I had a patient a few years back, Emily, who came to me with a complaint. She was married to one of my former patients, and she told me, "It's not fair. Spencer and I both had braces as teenagers, and Spencer went to you, and I went to another orthodontist. But Spencer's teeth are still beautiful, and he's having no problems. My teeth are crooked, my jaws are killing me, and I've had headaches ever since I was a teenager."

We began by addressing Emily's TMJ issues, which were the cause of her headaches and pain, then we corrected her bite. Some expansion of her upper jaw was necessary, as were some outpatient procedures. Had this been addressed when she was a teen, it would have been much simpler—but we were able to give her a beautiful smile and a healthy, comfortable bite. She hasn't had a headache since, and told me that it changed her life. I hear that all the time, and making that difference for my patients has been a personal goal of mine, one that I've pursued throughout my career.

Before I became an orthodontist, I was a dentist for six years, so I had been trained in how bites fit together properly. From my perspective as a dentist, I'd see my patients come back from the orthodontist, and more often than not I was disappointed in the results. Even though the cosmetic results looked good, I could see that the patient was left with a bad bite, and I knew sooner or later that would create havoc for them.

Why weren't orthodontists more conscious of the need for a healthy bite? I was complaining about it one day to one of my colleagues, and he said, "Well, do something about it. Be an orthodontist."

And I thought, "You know what? You're right." That's when I decided I was going to learn how to do this better. That became my "why".

The techniques needed to make the kinds of bite corrections I do are not taught in ordinary residencies, so I went for extra training over the course of two years at The Roth Williams Center for Functional Occlusion. They treated patients with TMJ—actively treated them, not just talked about it in lecture and theory. It was fascinating, and I signed on for more courses. I didn't have two nickels to rub together, but I was spending tens of thousands of dollars and taking weeks at a time away for my practice to get better at what I did, because I felt like my patients deserved that.

It was Dr. Ron Roth who pioneered the adoption of the techniques and tools of restorative dentists and applied them to orthodontics. It was a controversial move, largely because it meant more complex and challenging work. It's a highly goal-oriented treatment, and we were given very specific techniques to get to those results.

I was fortunate enough to study at The Roth Williams Center for Functional Occlusion with some of the finest orthodontists in the world. At the end of the training I was able to take what I'd learned and use it to not only create beautiful, cosmetic results for my patients but also to correct the kinds of bite dysfunctions that so rarely get fixed.

Why doesn't every orthodontist do this? It's expensive to learn, for one thing, and takes time and work to master the tools and techniques. It troubles me that, as a profession, we're more apt to put research into finding reasons to not do these kinds of things than we are in acknowledging their importance and learning how to do them. That makes me the odd man out as a practitioner. But I've seen too many cases like Bob's and Emily's to write off the lifelong issues that a bad bite can create.

In Chapter 5, I'll go into a more specifics about the proprietary techniques we use exclusively at White Orthodontics to make sure that the orthodontic treatment we provide is "Done Right"!

Chapter One

Why Is My Child's Smile So Important?

IF YOU ARE WEIGHING the yes/no and now/later decisions of orthodontic care or braces, you'll be trying to decide just how important or unimportant it really is.

Some parents feel "looks aren't everything." Some think their kid should just be tough-minded about this and not overly sensitive. Some may not have had orthodontic care when they were children and think, *Hey, I turned out just fine. I have a great spouse, a good career, friends—so what's the big deal?*

But that was then. This is *now*: the age of social media.

Social shaming and bullying is a lot worse, a lot more common, and a lot more persistent than when you were a kid. Teen suicide is on the rise, and such suicides share one thing in common: shocked and bewildered parents who could not conceive of their child ending his own life. Sure, they might've noticed he was a *little* depressed. They knew he was being bullied and spending more time home, alone, not leaving his room, but geez, he *is* a teenager, after all. What once was a few days or weeks of misery contained in the cafeteria with a few bullies is now endless, expansive, and broadcast online to everybody. Behind a computer screen, it can get far nastier than most would dare in person. Sometimes, kids bully each other for no reason, being a buck-toothed girl or a boy with gaps in between their teeth is enough to exacerbate the situation.

Signs Your Child May Be Being Bullied

- decrease in self-esteem

- not wanting to go to school

- skipping school

- injuries they can't explain

- self-destructive behaviors (e.g., harming themselves)

- declining school grades

- sleep difficulties

- loss of interest in schoolwork or activities

- sudden loss of friends or avoiding social groups

- changes in eating habits

A straight, clean and healthy smile can not only give your child the confidence she needs to embrace her true worth, but can also pave the way toward easier socialization at school, church, or during extracurricular activities. Do your child a favor and talk about her smile and how it might be affecting her.

Beyond that, there's a life ahead of your child. Going to junior high with crooked teeth and a humiliating smile is one thing. Hey, plenty of kids are going to school *without shoes* for heaven's sake. But going to college admission interviews, packing up and heading off to college, going to job interviews, trying to fit into new and anxiety-rich environments at a faraway college or new workplace with a bad smile—and maybe unavoidable bad breath with it—and daytime headaches from nighttime teeth-grinding is a lot more serious.

This isn't *just* a cosmetic issue. Misaligned, crooked teeth equal *significant* medical problems.

Poorly aligned teeth can produce chronic headaches and migraines, contribute to digestive problems because of the inability to properly chew foods, and make getting a decent night's sleep impossible. Perhaps the most dangerous of all: it can foster gum disease. Gum disease has absolute links to diabetes, heart disease, strokes and dementia, as well as, of course, the loss of natural teeth altogether. Orthodontic corrections later in adult life are more difficult; they can be painful, require time off work, and at best, they'll just be embarrassing. *Invisible braces aren't really totally invisible, and you're thirty-eight? Forty-four? Fifty-one? C'mon.*

Uncorrected mouth problems and misaligned teeth make for strangely stretched gums inevitably destined to separate from teeth. This could allow "pockets" for infections and periodontal disease to arise and turn into *very* difficult, painful, and costly problems late in life.

In the teenage years, failure to spend even $5,000 can easily create a $50,000 full mouth restoration case at age forty or fifty, or embarrassing, health-compromising removal of all teeth and use of dentures at age sixty.

Gum disease is serious business. It worsens the risks of and heightens dangers from diabetes, heart disease, strokes, and dementia. Ignoring preteen or teen teeth misalignment may virtually guarantee adult medical problems. If there is a genetic history of any of these medical problems I just named, you only worsen the odds of your son or daughter suffering from them by ignoring or postponing needed orthodontic treatment.

Aside from impacting health, a poorly aligned smile can significantly impact your child's comfort. Headaches, toothaches, sinus problems, dry mouth, snoring, drooling, bad breath, and insomnia are all symptoms of a smile that isn't straight, jaws that aren't aligned, or teeth that are too close together or not quite close enough. Oftentimes, however, the mouth is the last place we check for signs of discomfort, loss of sleep, or even a simple headache.

If your child's pediatrician can't figure out why she's not sleeping well or experiencing headaches or even insomnia for which there seems to be no cause, a simple thirty-minute exam at your local orthodontist could provide a clear solution in no time!

Here is what I'm told by an awful lot of parents:

"I had wonderful parents, *but* I sure wish they had found a way to afford the braces I needed and gotten me the care I needed when I was a kid, so I didn't grow up to have this bad smile my whole life."

And what I hear from almost every adult patient getting orthodontic treatment and braces is:

"I had wonderful parents, *but* I sure wish they had found a way to afford the braces I needed and gotten me the care

I needed when I was a kid, so I didn't grow up to have this bad smile my whole life *and have all these problems now.*"

Is this how you want your daughter or son talking about you ten, twenty, or thirty years from now? Is this how you want them remembering their childhood? Your parenting?

If that sounds pretty damned pushy, I admit: it is. I kept it in the book for the very simple reason that this is *truly* what I have heard so much over the years, and I am sincere about letting you reflect on it. All parents want to do the right thing. They don't want to let their children down in any way, and I'm sure you don't either.

You know, parents just about kill themselves over their kids' college, trying their best to guide the decision, trekking around the country on campus visits, worrying over campus culture, or taking on *serious* debt. Every parent understands what many kids can't— that it's not about the few years of college but rather the forty or fifty years afterward.

I assure you, this is the same. It's not about the bad, humiliating smile and bad bite transformed now, for high school. It's about the many, many years to come. They really can't appreciate that now, but *you* can.

No parent wants their child to suffer, either from teeth that actually hurt, headaches you can't explain, insomnia that affects their daily life, or insecurity your child may be feeling because of a crooked or oversized smile. The fact is, your child's formative years are actually the most sensitive for his or her teeth. Now is the time to pay close attention to your child's smile, behavior, peer relationships, and confidence level.

If any or all are lacking, a qualified orthodontist may help give you and your child the peace of mind you both crave.

The Top Five Reasons People Avoid Seeing the Orthodontist

1. **Patients are afraid it's going to hurt.** Pain is the number-one reason most people avoid going to the orthodontist. However, modern technology—and choosing the right orthodontist—can ensure that your child enjoys a pain-free orthodontic experience.

2. **Patients are afraid it's going to cost too much.** Not only are most orthodontic procedures more affordable than ever, but insurance, payment plans, and a variety of other financing options make this all but a moot point for most of my patients. Remember, orthodontists aren't in this to get rich, they're here to make sure your child's teeth, smile, and jaw are aligned to make his or her life better—period! We're not going to let something like price get in the way of creating a better, safer, healthier smile for your child.

3. **Patients are afraid it's going to take too long / they're going to miss too much school or work.** Regardless of the type of orthodontic procedure your child needs, time is of the essence. Modern technology and ease of access allows us to work around your child's school schedule with minimal absences. After initial visits, and barring the actual procedure itself, most visits and/or adjustments are routine and can take anywhere from fifteen to forty-five minutes.

4. **Patients do not see the need to take action.** Eroding, crooked, or unaligned smiles can take

time to happen, but the time to act is now. Orthodontic irregularities don't just heal on their own or disappear if you ignore them. Your child's smile and overall dental health are too important to ignore out of questions of pain, convenience, or even price.

5. **Patients have been treated in the past with an attitude of indifference.** Let's face it, not all doctors are created equal. Every profession has its "bad apples," and to say dentistry is the exception would be to write fiction instead of fact. There is no room for indifference when it comes to your child's healthcare. Find an orthodontic specialist that offers not only state of the art technology for your child, but state of the art service as well. Orthodontic specialists know what it's like to sit in the chair, and should provide every opportunity for patients, especially our younger patients, to feel comfortable, safe, and secure in our care.

Call us at **804-704-8374** or go to **SmileRichmond.com** to schedule your own Customized White Orthodontics Smile Analysis.

Chapter Two

Why Do Kids Need Braces?

ARE BRACES SOMETHING CREATED by orthodontists to make money, like Disney and their extra-charge FastPass? Was it a conspiracy from the very start?

Then and now, there may be some overprescribing and premature prescribing by some doctors. There are bad apples in every orchard. And you know the adage: if all he's got is a hammer, everything (and everybody) looks like a nail.

But there is a very legitimate, clinically documented, and 90 percent of the time, clearly visible reason why some kids, as young as eight, *need* orthodontic treatment and care: malocclusion.

Malocclusion is mostly genetic, so if your daughter or son has it, blame their grandparents. It's a fancy-pants term for all things related to misaligned teeth—teeth growing angled, crooked, and into a too-crowded space. It can be a single tooth, a few teeth, or the whole mouth. As I said, it is mostly hereditary, and your kids didn't get to pick their parents out of a Barbie catalog. There can be other causes too, like early, premature loss of primary teeth, chronic thumb-sucking, or even an accident that seemed to leave no lasting effect at its moment in time.

If your child is suffering from any, several, or all of the following early indicators of malocclusion, consider having them addressed by an orthodontic specialist sooner rather than later:

- **Crossbites**: A crossbite occurs when the jaw deviates to one side with an improper fit of the upper and lower teeth from left to right or front to back. Crossbites can lead to worn and chipped teeth, jaw pain, and asymmetric growth of the jaws. Left untreated, the crossbite will require more extensive treatment later in life and significant jaw surgery in the most-severe cases.

- **Thumb-sucking**: Thumb-sucking habits beginning at the age of seven or older should be corrected immediately in order to prevent severe jaw and tooth alignment problems.

- **Miscellaneous concerns**: There are several associated issues you should also be looking for as soon as your child turns seven in order to intervene early, including the following:

  ▫ permanent teeth that are growing into the wrong spots

  ▫ severely protruded front teeth at risk for injury or causing teasing at school

  ▫ severe crowding with permanent teeth erupting into poor-quality gum tissue

With any of these situations, we can discuss the pros and cons of early intervention and treatment versus waiting until all the permanent teeth are in for braces. If you are anxious about the appearance of your child's teeth or your child is self-conscious about his or her appearance, early treatment might be the best choice. Not only are most orthodontic problems more difficult to correct later, but self-image and personality inhibition can be hard for a person to leave behind. However, if your child is extremely resistant to braces or is not mature enough to be trusted to care for them, delay may be the better choice. In that case, regularly scheduled orthodontic checkups will be necessary.

Having malocclusion does *not* guarantee a child will need braces. Frankly, this is what worries me about nonspecialists like family dentists substituting themselves for orthodontists, and parents letting it happen. They may easily miss an early diagnosis of malocclusion, when it could have been treated without braces. Or they may leap to braces as the only way to treat all malocclusion. Either way, you and your child lose.

The first question, then, is: does your daughter or son have or show all the signs they are going to have malocclusion? Second, if so, what—of numerous options—should be done about it? Third, when?

To have all these questions answered early, the first full orthodontic exam should occur early in a child's life. I recommend seven or eight, no later than nine, especially if there is family history of malocclusion. With early and periodic exams by an orthodontic specialist, you may avoid your child's need for braces and/or you may prevent years of suffering and embarrassment related to their teeth and smile.

Waiting will have very serious consequences, often requiring more treatment and higher costs later in life. What most parents fail to realize is that these treatment problems are urgent and should be treated as such. If that ship has sailed, the next best time for a full orthodontic exam is tomorrow at three o'clock.

If your son or daughter does need braces—now or at some predictable future time—the outcome of the exam can lead to *sensible* decisions. If not now, treatment to prevent the need can begin, and also, you can begin saving money for braces or other procedures if necessary later on in your child's life. There is no tooth fairy coming to leave a few thousand dollars underneath his pillow or yours. But if the need must be met three years from now, skipping one Starbucks run a week for those three years can make a hefty dent in the bill to come. Utilizing a Health Savings Account or Flex Spending Account can help, as well. How to fund orthodontic treatment is discussed later in the book.

Let me be emphatically clear. I am *not* in the business of putting braces on any child who doesn't need braces. My office is *not* a braces store. I'm in the business of helping kids and families get the right orthodontic treatment if any is needed, get the right braces if any are needed, and have as perfect a smile and as few oral health problems as possible. I make sure my patients are informed—that's why I wrote this book. In my office, you're never told what to do. You're provided with real information, no medical jargon, plain English, "reasons why," and options. You probably know the term "God complex," referring to a person who acts like he's God—imperious, brusque, and deliberately intimidating to squash questions. You will *not* get that kind of treatment here, from me or anyone on my team.

Kids do need braces, but not all kids and certainly not the same braces for all. Some kids are better served by other orthodontic treatments instead of or before braces. We will collaborate, you and I, to figure out what is or isn't needed and what options are best if there is a need for your child.

Call us at **804-704-8374** or go to **SmileRichmond.com** to schedule your own Customized White Orthodontics Smile Analysis.

"We love Dr. White and his entire staff! They are awesome—always so friendly and helpful. But most importantly, Dr. White was able to help our daughter avoid jaw surgery in spite of lost time spent with another orthodontist!"

- A. CISZAK

Chapter Three

Why Not Just a Dentist?
Why an Orthodontist?

YOU UNDOUBTEDLY ALREADY have a dentist.

Gee, isn't seeing an orthodontist going to cost a lot more?

I'm busy. More appointments?

Do I really need to get orthodontic checkups for my kids?

Don't worry, these are all reasonable questions! It is true that, today, quite a few dentists dance over into our territory, and although they're *not* permitted to claim they're the same as orthodontists or provide orthodontic treatment (beware of any who do), they're able to do things like provide Invisalign and other braces. This can be confusing. Here are the facts.

All orthodontists are dentists and we all graduate from the same dental schools. True enough. But that's where it stops for dentists. Orthodontists go to school for an additional two to three years to become credentialed specialists at diagnosing and providing the best treatment for conditions like:

- difficulties chewing or biting
- constant biting into the cheek, gums, or roof of the mouth
- teeth that meet abnormally or don't meet at all
- teeth grinding or clenching
- crowded, misplaced, or blocked out teeth
- early or late loss of teeth
- teeth grown in badly
- teeth that protrude
- embarrassing personal appearance due to teeth
- facial imbalances
- teeth or jaw misalignment, TMJ
- chronic headaches and migraine
- poor sleep
- speech difficulties (that may never be outgrown or may develop later)

These are *not* dental care issues. They are orthodontic issues.

For *some* things, a generalist or jack-of-all-trades will do. For other things, you know it's smart to seek out the best specialist you can afford. For example, if all your income is in a single W-2 from one employer and you have simple, ordinary deductions, getting your taxes prepared for the cheapest fee at the seasonal H&R Block office that opens up in your neighborhood shopping center is probably fine. But if you have W-2, 1099, and investment income from real estate, depreciation on real estate in several states, own stocks, and you raise iguanas as a money hobby, you're going to get yourself a really good accountant, probably a CPA. If you need the simplest will, leaving everything first to spouse or second to daughter may be okay. But if you are of some means and have several children and maybe also grandchildren as well as charities, you're going to need to see an *estate planning* attorney, not just any attorney—though they all went to the same law schools—but *a specialist in estate planning*.

This is no different.

There are a few things to keep in mind when differentiating between a general dentist and an orthodontic specialist.

First, generalists, or jacks-of-all-trades, tend to work with one-size-fits-all, off-the-rack, standardized solutions. They may be limited to doing only what the computer dictates that they do, without bringing expertise and expert judgment to bear. They're often working with products from only one provider, without being able to select from a full range of options that would work best for you. Specialists, instead, tend to individually and carefully diagnose needs and provide personalized solutions.

Second, generalists and their use of inexpertly applied, standardized solutions tend to be cheaper than the fees of a specialist, but that also places economic pressure on them to do the treatment as quickly and simply as possible, because they've "cut it thin."

In this case, it's worth remembering that the treatment provided has permanent, lifelong, and life-impacting consequences. This concerns your health, future dental or jaw alignment or misalignment issues affecting quality of sleep (which can affect weight, even onset and management of type 2 diabetes and heart disease), as well as self-esteem and social and career success.

> **General Dentist.** A general dentist gives routine checkups, preventative measures, cleans teeth, and fixes cavities. They may not start seeing children until they are seven to ten years old.
>
> **Pediatric Dentist.** A pediatric dentist has two to three years of specialized education beyond dental school. They specialize in providing dental care to children and adolescents, offering checkups, preventative measures, cleanings, and cavities.
>
> **Orthodontist.** An orthodontist has two to three years of specialized education beyond dental school and is an expert at straightening teeth and aligning the jaws. They assess patients and determine the best treatment routes and procedures that need to be taken.

If you can, you want to choose an orthodontist for orthodontic care.

You may ask, *how do I know my doctor is an orthodontist?* It's a good question and a critical one to ask as you seek additional treatment for your child's dental issues.

Only orthodontists can belong to the American Association of Orthodontists (AAO). If you're looking for a local orthodontist, go online and visit **www.braces.org** to find a specialist in your area. This website features not only a searchable database of orthodontists but educational tips, answers and resources to help you on your quest for your child's healthiest smile!

Alternatively, you can ask your doctor if he or she has completed a two- to three-year residency in orthodontics and check with your state dental board to follow up on his reply. Dentists and orthodontists in most states will be registered differently with the dental board.

Do your homework; be a "dental detective" while on the hunt for such vital information. Look for the words "dental specialist in orthodontics," or ask your general dentist for a referral to a specialist. In urban and suburban areas, it will take minimal effort to find a specialist. In more remote, rural locations, your search might take you to another city or town. Don't be afraid to ask your dentist if an orthodontist travels to your town every month to see patients. There's a chance an orthodontist from a larger city comes to your town and works out of another dental office once or twice per month. Looking around can save valuable driving time and money.

One note: there is no disrespect between orthodontists and dentists. As a matter of fact, many orthodontic patients are referred by their dentists. These are great, capable, and caring professionals who know where their expertise begins and ends, and who do not let ego or income opportunity step in front of what they know is best for their patients. Just as the family doctor refers his patients with possible or significant heart disease issues to a cardiologist, and if need be, the cardiologist refers to a surgeon, the best dentists refer patients with orthodontic needs to orthodontists. Orthodontists are required to take two to three years of university education beyond dental school and additional continuing clinical education every year. They must also invest in state-of-the-art technology for their offices (not found in dental offices)—*all for a good reason.*

Even though we orthodontists have the education and training to perform general dentist procedures, we don't. We specialize.

Call us at **804-704-8374** or go to **SmileRichmond.com** to schedule your own Customized White Orthodontics Smile Analysis.

"The process has been smooth, fast and easy. Dr. White and his staff have been so helpful and supportive. We did con-sultations with several orthodontists but chose Dr. White because his plan was more com-prehensive, long term and well thought out."

- K. SHIELDS

Chapter Four

Choose a Highly Successful Orthodontist

WHY IS THAT IMPORTANT? Wouldn't you get a "better deal" from one barely getting the light bill paid? Maybe. But an overeager orthodontist—or maybe more so, an overeager dentist eager to do braces—might be seeing needs that are more urgent than they really are.

What are some good clues to selecting a great orthodontist?

I've got two: his practice is busy.

I assure you, the ability of advertising to attract orthodontic patients is limited and it's expensive. When you see a really, really busy practice, there are probably a whole lot of patient referrals, and neither kids nor parents enthusiastically refer if they feel they were lied to or treated badly, put in pain, or wound up with results nothing like the digital future-photo they were shown. And they probably wouldn't come to that practice if they had to keep coming back to "fix a few things," or were overcharged. Parents tell parents about great orthodontic practices because we earned their trust and because their kids keep thanking them.

I keep my office very busy. Yes, we advertise. But mostly, these practices thrive by patient referrals. Not that I would anyway, but I don't need to goad you into more and more expensive care than your son's or daughter's situation requires for the best outcome. I don't need to "sell" four more sets of braces this month to win a cruise from the manufacturer—and yes, that stuff goes on in some practices. There's an old cartoon from the *Wall Street Journal* with a bunch of executives in a boardroom at a conference table, one hollering, "Ethics? Ethics? We can't afford ethics!"

This is a business, a business built on ethics and earned trust. And you do *not* just need a doctor to install braces; you need a trustworthy advisor.

The other clue: a great orthodontist is *not* cheap.

Our fees are calculated to allow for "Cadillac + Care" in every respect, to put no downward financial pressure on how we care for patients and parents, and to *never* cut corners or take shortcuts. We *never* use any material that is "probably good enough."

If I were you, I'd worry if I could find an orthodontist that is a lot cheaper anywhere else. If you do find one, know this: behind closed doors they're probably asking, "Can we do this cheaper?" Is *that* the question you want discussed back there, at every step of your child's treatment?

This isn't even like Botox. It's more like cosmetic surgery. There's a science and an art to this. My orthodontists and my staff are all highly trained to produce state-of-the-art outcomes, nothing less. The doctor makes a difference. That's why I tell everybody to get a highly successful orthodontist.

The Most Important Things You Should Know *Before* Choosing Your Orthodontist

This is something you want to be sure about.

I've just suggested one big consideration: a very successful practice. Here are eleven more.

1. Are they a specialist?

Orthodontists are dentists who take on several extra years of special training in order to straighten teeth, usually by affixing braces to the patient's teeth. You might say we specialize in smiles. Orthodontists also perform dentofacial orthopedics. This is a fancy way to describe how we normalize the structure of a patient's jaw bones in order to repair any imbalance in their face. All orthodontists are dentists, but only 6 percent of dentists are orthodontists. Look for the seal of the American Association of Orthodontists (AAO). Only orthodontic specialists can belong to the AAO.

2. Are they trained to treat TMJ disorders?

Over 65 percent of people, young and old, suffer from a TMJ or jaw joint disorder. Symptoms may range from jaw clicking or popping and headaches to jaw locking, ringing in the ears, vertigo and neck aches. The majority of these people have a malocclusion (or bad bite) that places undue stress on the jaw joints, jaw muscles, and the teeth and their supporting structures such as the gums and bone, creating an imbalance. Most jaw joint problems develop over time; many of the early signs and symptoms can be overlooked by an untrained dentist or orthodontist. Most orthodontists focus primarily on aligning the teeth and improving the smile. Some even talk about correcting the bite, but have had minimal training and do very little to actually correct the bite properly.

So far, I've helped thousands of people who suffered from TMJ achieve a beautiful smile, and more importantly, a healthy, "pain free" bite. In fact, most of my patients are referred to me because of their TMJ problems. Fortunately, I have incorporated the same principles and techniques that's used to help TMJ patients for my routine orthodontic patients to help them avoid a future full of expensive, painful and sometimes debilitating jaw joint disorders.

If you or someone you know is suffering from a jaw joint disorder or may have TMJ, please contact our office for a complimentary TMJ screening and bite evaluation.

3. Do they take a holistic approach?

Most people imagine straight teeth and a great-looking smile when they think about orthodontics and that, of course, is a great reason to wear braces or invisalign. However, you may be surprised to learn that an improper bite can cause a myriad of problems beyond a basic aesthetic appearance, including crooked teeth, premature tooth wear, gum recession, headaches, jaw clicking, and in extreme cases, even tooth loss.

If you or someone you know has a bad bite, just straightening the teeth will rarely correct these problems. The health of the head and neck area is determined by a delicate balance between several "systems." These systems include the muscles and the soft tissues of the face, the airway, the jaw joints, the shape and alignment of the upper and lower jaws, and—last but not least—the alignment and fit of the teeth, otherwise know as the bite. As you search for the "right" orthodontist for you or a loved one, you should consider these two important questions regarding the orthodontist and his or her philosophy:

- Does the orthodontist take into account how their treatment plan will establish harmony between these systems and create balance between the bite and a stable jaw joint position?

- Does the orthodontist take a proactive early treatment approach to use a younger patient's natural growth in order to decrease the severity of the orthodontic problem and, thereby, lessening the chance of permanent tooth removal or jaw surgery?

As you may have guessed, the answer to both of these questions for the treatment we provide at White Orthodontics is a resounding "Yes"! Every patient receives an in-depth evaluation, including a 3-D airway and jaw alignment analysis, a state-of-the-art jaw joint assessment, and a treatment plan to enhance the soft tissues and muscles of the head and neck. Our treatment plan will even consider how a patient's face and smile may change as they age.

4. Do they treat children and adults?

Orthodontics is not just for kids! While the majority of our patients are kids or young adults, we do help many adults transform their smiles, too. It is important that your orthodontist can treat patients of all ages. In fact, 30 percent of the orthodontic patients we see in our office are adults. Many adults are finding out how a healthy and attractive smile is important to their health and the way they feel a bout themselves. Others choose to avoid a lifetime of crooked teeth for health concerns or problems with their bite that can lead to premature tooth wear, gum recession or TMJ problems. With today's discreet treatment options, adults and teens are able to get a beautiful smile without wearing metal braces!

5. Do they provide the first visit free of charge?

Most orthodontists offer free examinations for new patients so you and your family can get expert advice about treatment needs, options, and timing before making this important investment.

During your first exam and consultation, be sure your questions are being answered, concerns addressed, and you are being educated about all of your treatment options.

Most orthodontists use digital x-rays during the initial exam. At White Orthodontics we include a digital 3-D scan which is much more detailed than a 2-D x-ray, giving us a significantly more com-prehensive view of the teeth and jaws, allowing me better accuracy in treatment planning.

There are also some orthodontists who won't give you a treatment fee until you've paid for orthodontic records. At our practice, should treatment be necessary, we will give you an exact fee and find a payment plan that will fit your budget prior to starting any treatment. We believe you shouldn't have to pay to find out how much your treatment will cost.

6. Do they offer a lifetime guarantee?

No matter which orthodontist you choose, ultimately you are not making a small investment in time or money. Because of this, don't you want to ensure your orthodontist is going to stand behind their treatment? Of course! At our practie your smile is protected by our lifetime guarantee!

After treatment, if your teeth shift or crowd, even if it's because you didn't wear your retainers, your re-treatment is completely free. No questions asked. We wouldn't have it any other way!

7. Are they using the latest technology and treatment options available?

Orthodontics today differs a great deal from years past. Computer-designed braces and wires dramatically increase the precision with which we move teeth and this, in turn, shortens treatment time. Tie-free braces systems have made treatment far more efficient and comfortable. Clear braces offer a cosmetically pleasing alternative, while Invisalign offers patients an entirely brace-free option. Did you know that Invisalign also has a special treatment system just for teens? At White Orthodontics, we guarantee that we can find the treatment option that will fit your lifestyle! We can even place braces behind your teeth!

In fact, I was the first orthodontist in Virginia to combine 3-D imagining with the amazing precision of SureSmile robotics. We also eliminated those "yucky" impress ions or molds of your teeth utilizing digital scanning and 3D model printing. Our patients love the ease and comfort of our "no mess" system!

8. Does their quoted fee include retainers?

Each orthodontic office has its own fee schedules, and doctors often charge differently for procedures. At White Orthodontics, our fee is "all inclusive" with no hidden charges. Throughout the orthodontic industry, it is common to find out about retainer fees and other hidden fees *after* you start treatment. Since you are reading this book, you can ask your orthodontist about their retainer costs and also if there are any other hidden fees.

In our practice, our "signature" is a custom-made, permanent retainer to help keep the lower front teeth straight for life. We also provide our patients with a clear top and bottom retainer to maintain their beautiful smiles.

9. Do they make you feel special and comfortable?

Regardless if you are reading this book for your own treatment or for your child's treatment, when you meet with your orthodontist, everyone should definitely feel comfortable throughout the process. The practice should strive to make you as comfortable as possible before, during, and after treatment.

Our practice always ensures your child feels special every time they visit. The majority of our team have children of their own, and since our team is so involved with children and young adults, we can emphathize, relate to them, and make them feel comfortable and extra special. Our Smile Rewards program is a positive reward system designed to help kids and young adults have fun and keep them engaged in their treatment.

10. Do they have a great reputation?

With the Internet today, it is extremely easy to pull up ratings and reviews from patients. Simply go to Google and search for orthodontist reviews and ratings in your town. You will see that we are 5-star rated on Google.

11. Are they flexible with payment options?

Once you are comfortable and know which orthodontist you want to treat you or your child, the next question typically is, "How much is this going to cost and how am I going to pay for this?"

At White Orthodontics, we will help you understand different payment options from maximizing the most insurance benefits to flex spending accounts to even interest-free payment plans. During the initial exam and complimentary consultation (a $298 value), we will answer all of your questions, including those about our typical cost of braces and the variety of payment options available.

How to Know What Questions to Ask

I've really thought through the questions most parents and patients have—not just the ones they ask, but the ones they don't. This book attempts to cover them all, but again, this is a *personal* matter. The best questions to ask are the ones that matter most to you and your child.

I hope not, but you may be in a position that absolutely requires you to get the minimum essential treatment for the lowest cost. If so, your most important questions are going to be about those kinds of options and about price, and nothing else.

If, however, you are able to make your decision about who you should trust with your child's oral health and smile by many factors, we've included a "What Is Most Important to You?" quiz from Excellence In Orthodontics on the following pages. As you'll see, there are fourteen different items to consider and rank in importance to you. Any can become the questions you ask me and my team or any other orthodontist.

Incidentally, Excellence In Orthodontics is a national organization for exceptionally successful orthodontists leading the field in both clinical and patient care and patient/parent (client) service excellence. We all subscribe to a pledge of very high standards and hold each other accountable. You can learn more at ExcellenceInOrthdontics.org.

If you have a specific question not answered anywhere in this book, or have a personal and confidential question, you can—with complete assurance of privacy and courtesy—email Info@SmileRichmond.com or call Dr. Paul R. White at 804-704-8374.

There is also a FAQ section at the back of this book.

Of course, a perfect opportunity to get questions answered—yours and your son's or daughter's—is at your exam appointment.

Call us at **804-704-8374** or go to **SmileRichmond.com** to schedule your own Customized White Orthodontics Smile Analysis.

What Is Most Important to You?

Directions: For each **Key Item** below, rank its importance to you from 1 to 5. Then check off whether each type of provider provides that item. When you're done with all 14 Key Items, add up your rankings and review what your final score means about choosing an orthodontist.

	Key Items to Consider in Selecting Your Orthodontist	Rank How Important Each Item Is to You in Selecting Your Orthodontist 1 – Not Important, 5 – Very Important	Check Off If Provided		
			White Orthodontics	Other Provider	Other Provider
1	Orthodontist and staff committed to expert, thorough diagnosis, and prescription of the best treatment plan customized for my son or daughter	1 2 3 4 5	✔		
2	Avoiding extractions (if possible)	1 2 3 4 5	✔		
3	Having esthetic options such as clear braces or aligners instead of metal braces	1 2 3 4 5	✔		
4	Having a healthy, pleasing smile that will last a lifetime and protect optimum dental health (not just having straightened teeth)	1 2 3 4 5	✔		
5	Pain-free treatment	1 2 3 4 5	✔		
6	Orthodontist utilizes the most modern, advanced, and proven technology, including computer-aided design and fitting	1 2 3 4 5	✔		
7	Orthodontists and team actively involved in continuing clinical education	1 2 3 4 5	✔		
8	Reducing treatment time to a minimum without compromising results (including total length of treatment term and number of office visits)	1 2 3 4 5	✔		
9	Availability of after-school or after-work appointment options	1 2 3 4 5	✔		
10	Treatment coordinator is knowledgeable about insurance coverage and is able to offer flexible payment plans	1 2 3 4 5	✔		
11	Getting the best overall value factoring in thorough diagnosis, customized care, and concern with lifetime health and well-being—not just the cheapest fee	1 2 3 4 5	✔		

12	Lifetime guarantee	1 2 3 4 5	✓		
13	Orthodontist and team committed to excellence in orthodontics and customer service for both patients and parents	1 2 3 4 5	✓		

Total of Your Rankings

What Your Score Means

50-70   There is no doubt. White Orthodontics is the right choice for you and your family! It is clear that you place a high value on a comprehensive, "best" approach.

43-49   You are probably also going to be happiest with White Orthodontics, rather than any other alternative. But this score suggests you aren't completely sure and have some unanswered questions or concerns. Your doctor and the practice's treatment coordinator want no lingering uncertainties on your part, and want to address any and every question. Don't keep anything to yourself. Please ask.

42 or less   Frankly, you may not value the advanced, sophisticated level of clinical care and customer service provided at White Orthodontics. Cost may be much more important to you than other factors, or very basic service may be all you feel you need. It's perfectly okay. If you choose to shop around, be sure to use this checklist in evaluating other options. Remember, you do want everything right the first time, and you want error-free orthodontics at a minimum.

"We completed treatment with another orthodontist, and we were so disappointed with the results that left my daughter's teeth in a very unattractive position. We came to Dr. White—and our daughter was resistant at first which was understandable as she was in eigth grade—but now she loves her new smile and is happy she got braces 'one more time' to get it right."

J. LIGGAN

Chapter Five

Braces Done Right, the First Time!

The costs of a bad bite

A lot of patients, many of who had braces years earlier, come to us suffering with headaches, neck aches and jaw pain. Some of them can barely open their mouths. Others can hardly chew. These issues all stem from what we call TMJ issues, the lack of proper balance between where the jaw hinges up in front of the ear, and the way in which the teeth mesh together. If those aren't properly coordinated, then the problems arise, because if the bite and jaw are out of balance, then the muscles of the jaw have to tighten and shift the jaw to make the teeth fit together. When the jaw shifts, the joint can become dislocated, and that's when problems occur.

Initially you may hear clicking or popping in your jaws. When the muscles have tightened up to pull the teeth together, they can fatigue, to the point it's hard to chew things—or in spasm, which is when you experience pain and headaches. That discomfort pushes you to change your posture, which in turn brings on neck aches. Your body will adapt to try and solve this imbalance, but not necessarily in a positive way.

These issues all stem from a bad bite created by the orthodontist's efforts to straighten the teeth with braces. With a child, the problems aren't necessarily noticeable, especially when you don't know how to look for them. It's when you get older, and you have less flexibility and you're putting more pressure on your bite that the symptoms start to appear.

As in Bob's case, a bad bite can also cause bone loss around the teeth, and periodontal disease has been linked to so many health problems in later life, including diabetes, stroke, and heart disease.

One patient had spent years suffering from headaches and had been in braces twice before she came to us. She had such a severe overbite that she needed to have her jaw lengthened with surgery to correct it. When it was done, she asked me, "Why didn't my other doctors just do this in the first place?" If they had, she'd not have had to go through all that suffering and expense.

Gum recession is another issue that can be linked to a bad bite. If your dentist sees your gums are receding, he's likely to blame it on brushing too hard—but the toothbrushes we use today are soft bristles with rounded ends, and most of us have learned to brush correctly. Again, the real culprit is your bad bite.

As with all issues caused by a bad bite, the most important part of the treatment is to make an accurate diagnosis, because as the Cheshire cat said, "If you don't know where you're going, any road will get you there." As a practitioner, you cannot see what you're not trained to see, so if you haven't had the extra training to understand the connection and understand the techniques, you're not going to be able to spot or address that underlying issue. I've taken what I learned from the best in this field, and combined it into a system of my own: Braces Done Right.

Diagnostics are key to getting braces done right

Treatment in our practice begins with advanced diagnostics, starting with a 3-D scan. We make the models of the patient's teeth and put it on a bite simulator (called an articulator). This lets us see the jaw joint position and how the teeth fit together with the jaw where it's supposed to be, because when you look at how a patient actually bites together habitually, these positions are often so different that the treatment plans will vary widely. That informs my treatment recommendations. Interestingly most of my staff that have previously worked for other orthodontists tell me, "At my old practice, the orthodontist never came into the room when we were checking the bite. We just had the patient bite down on a piece of wax," and that's standard orthodontic practice. In contrast, we make a registration of the bite with the jaw where it's supposed to be, which is one of the things I was trained to do at the Roth Williams Center. When a patient has TMJ problems, we also do a series of specialized jaw joint x-rays—again, an extra step that very few orthodontists take, but one which can make a huge difference in your results.

Armed with this information, we create the treatment plan. Other orthodontists might examine the same patient and simply recommend braces, but as I've said, you can't see what you haven't been trained to spot, and braces alone can't correct a serious bite problem. Precision in how treatment is applied is critical to success; specific adjustments have to be made during the course of treatment to achieve optimal results. Again, we're told as orthodontists that all we have to do is put these braces on with a straight wire, and everything will magically turn out where it's supposed to be. Unfortunately, too many orthodontists don't get the braces on where they belong in the first place.

I use a technique in which I first put the braces on a model of my patient's teeth. That gives me time to think about and adjust where I want each brace to be, and to make sure it gets in its ideal position. Then we transfer that positioning from the model to the mouth, using an athletic mouth guard material as a kind of mold. The precision of this process is important, because every time you move something, there's a chance for error.

In the planning stages of treatment, we also take into consideration the fourth dimension of time: what's the patient's face going to look like thirty years from now? As you get older, your face tends to collapse in, and you tend to get those creases at the corners of the mouth and up from your nose to the corners of the mouth. The wider and fuller your smile is, the less of that you get when you're older. Often expansion of the upper jaw is part of the treatment program. Not only is it healthier, it makes the bite fit better, and it gives you a more natural, wider-looking smile that helps support your face as you age. I compare it to doing a facelift on a teenager that kicks in thirty years later, because we're creating the structure that will support the face as it ages. Obviously, that's not on the teenager's mind when they're getting braces, but it's on mine.

When we're about three quarters of the way through treatment, we take an extraordinary "extra" step to make sure we deliver the exceptional results that our patients deserve. We make new models of the patient's straightened teeth, then put these models on the bite simulator to check the jaw position and the bite to assess the degree of improvement. We then make whatever changes are necessary to continue to correct them. Then, we check the jaw joint position as well as the condition of the teeth themselves. Finally, and most importantly, I shape and form custom-made wires that are inserted into the braces that will move all of the teeth to their final, ideal positions. I am amazed that I've never heard of another orthodontist taking this necessary step. I realize it involves extra effort and expense, but it's the key to achieving a beautiful, and more importantly, healthy smile.

Once we've got the bite corrected and the back teeth set, and the width and balance of the smile are right, we remove the braces. Even without the braces, I can still make subtle, but precise changes to the angles of the front teeth by using a series of aligners—we call it "Clear Finish." We use a proprietary system where we do a 3-D optical scan of the teeth to create a digital model of the patient's teeth. Then, on a computer, I move these digital teeth to an absolutely perfect bite and, subsequently, we make a series of clear aligners designed to achieve that result. Usually it's just a few aligners, and they're strictly to finalize and perfect the bite, so the back and front teeth are touching like they're supposed to. Again, this isn't standard operating procedure in orthodontics generally, but it should be.

Finally, we adjust the biting surface of the teeth, because if teeth don't have the proper shape, even well done orthodontics is only going to get you in the ballpark, so you have to fine-tune the shape of the teeth so that all their hills and valleys fit together properly. Teeth have to mesh like the gears of a bike, and if they don't have the appropriate shape, they can't fit together correctly. If they don't fit together correctly, as soon as you bite, you're going to start putting undesirable pressure on the teeth, and that's when they'll start to crowd up again.

When treatment is finished, you've got to be able to maintain what you've accomplished. Otherwise, you've spent a lot of time and money for nothing. A healthy bite is the best retainer in the world, but I do provide custom-made retainers for my patients using the same kind of modeling process, just as added insurance.

Much of what we do is done behind the scenes. This means patients don't have to be in the chair for hours, but they still get the precision they need. It's a demanding way to practice, requiring extra time and effort, but my patients see the results even if they don't see the work. Too often people wind up with beautiful smiles but bad bites, or good bites but not great looking smiles. My philosophy is that you deserve both, and that can't be achieved with a quick fix.

Airway Issues

Your orthodontist might not be the first person you think of if your child snores, has been diagnosed with ADHD, or wets the bed, but in fact, all of these issues can be a result of childhood sleep apnea or sleep disordered breathing (SDB). The same 3-D imaging technology we use to make "virtual" molds of your teeth can also be an important diagnostic tool for airway issues.

With the advent of 3-D imaging, we're able to go beyond the 2-D view that x-rays gave us. When you take a flat, 2-D x-ray, all the structures on the right side are superimposed over the top of the left side, and it's hard to tell what's what. 3-D provides a highly detailed and accurate image, and it also allows us to diagnose problems with the patient's airway. Every child that visits our office gets an airway screening, because if you're not breathing properly, it can create a whole range of health problems, behavioral issues, and even developmental and learning issues. Sleep apnea is generally associated with adults, but it often starts in childhood, and if we can diagnose it, we can treat it early. Adults with sleep apnea are far more likely to get heart disease, diabetes, stroke and other life-threatening health conditions, so clearly the sooner it's addressed, the better the outcome for your growing child. Children with sleep apnea caused by constricted airways are often misdiagnosed as being hyperactive, and dosed with powerful and unnecessary drugs that don't address the unseen root cause.

The airway is formed by the palate, the back of the throat, the tongue, the tonsils and the adenoids. When your tongue can't go up and forward where it's supposed to be, because the palate's too narrow, it pushes the tongue back and down. When the tongue gets forced backward, that can block the airway. One of the most effective orthodontic treatments for an airway problem is expanding the upper jaw. Widening the palate creates room that lets the tongue move forward into its proper position. If the problem is caused by enlarged tonsils or adenoids, which are obstructing the airway, the usual treatment is to remove them. But research shows that that this treatment is actually 60 percent to 70 percent more effective on a growing child if it's done in combination with expanding the upper jaw.

Catching this problem in time to prevent or correct the issues it creates is literally life-changing for a lot of children—and potentially life-saving for them as adults.

The challenge of choosing your orthodontist

If you're reading this book, chances are you're about to choose an orthodontist for yourself or your child. The problem for most consumers is they don't have enough information to make a good decision. And if we've got dentists that have been to four years of college and four years of dental school and still don't understand it, how can a consumer who hasn't had any dental training make a good decision?

That's why it's so important to me to educate people, show them why the conditions exist, and explain what needs to be done to correct them. Too often, the ones who understand the best are those who've had treatment somewhere else and now need to be retreated because it wasn't done correctly in the first place. They always say, "I wish I'd come to you first." And the challenge to the consumer is that, until there's a problem, you don't know that something's wrong.

As one of my former patients, Adair, who now lives in New York City, recently told me, "Every time I go to the dentist, they tell me that my bite is perfect and my smile is incredible. When they ask me who did my braces, I proudly reply, 'Dr. Paul White in Richmond, VA.'" That's the kind of result you deserve. Take the time to do your due diligence before you make this very important decision with life-long implications. If done properly, orthodontic treatment is one of the best investments you can make for you or your child which will pay huge benefits years after the braces are removed.

Call us at **804-704-8374** or go to **SmileRichmond.com** to schedule your own Customized White Orthodontics Smile Analysis.

"I am a dental hygienist and I highly recommend Dr. White. I tell my patients and friends about him. I was told by another dental hygienist that her office definitely sends their 'hardest' cases to Dr. White. I believe all cases should go to him!"

- B. MERGENMEIER, RDH

Chapter Six

What Can I Expect at the Initial Consultation and Exam?

MANY QUESTIONS SURROUND YOUR first visit to a new orthodontist, not the least of which is the subject of this particular chapter: *what will happen at the initial consultation?*

To answer this very common question, and perhaps several others you might not even realize you need answering yet, let me walk you through the typical first office visit, from the initial appointment forward. Your first appointment is scheduled following your initial phone call to your orthodontist's office.

1. **On arrival at the office, you will be greeted by one of our certified treatment coordinators**. She or he is fully prepared to make everything from the first appointment to an entire treatment program go smoothly for you and your child. Your treatment coordinator will manage your relationship with us, from appointment scheduling for your convenience to answering questions.

At the initial visit, your treatment coordinator will review your child's patient information and health history and and/or any appearance concerns with you.

This interview and required-by-law paperwork doesn't take long. You may also be asked to view, with your son or daughter, a pre-exam video to educate you on some of the important issues to consider with orthodontics.

2. **Next, Dr. White will conduct a "Customized Smile Analysis,"** the most complete and thorough orthodontic exam, including teeth, gums, mouth, jaws, and face. A state-of-the-art 3-D digital scan of the teeth and jaws will be made. Molds or an optical scan of the teeth may also be made if treatment is needed.

Usually that same day, your orthodontist will present his or her "report of findings"—a "show-n-tell," in plain English (not medical jargon), of the full state of your child's teeth, gums, mouth and jaws, and a diagnosis of any present or anticipated problems that should get orthodontic treatment. If treatment should occur, your orthodontist will present recommendations and options. This will be an individualized, personalized plan of treatment, not "braces in a box, off the shelf." By this report of findings, you will know:

- what teeth or jaw misalignment or other problems exist or are developing

- what the health and appearance ramifications are of not intervening with treatment

- if braces are needed now or later and which type of braces will be best in your situation

- what the complete treatment program will consist of, such as braces, number of appointments, and average time of each office visit

- what results will be achieved at the end of treatment

3. **All your questions will be answered**. There are no dumb or embarrassing questions. Every single one of my patients has a question, simple or complex! We do *not* want you or your son or daughter just nodding, then later wondering, "What did he mean by *that?*" or saying, "I wish I'd asked about …" This is *not* one of those "I'm the doctor—trust me—just do what I say because I said so" offices. Most questions will have been answered by the pre-exam video, other literature provided to you, this book, and your orthodontist's report of findings, but it's a lot to take in. So, any and all questions you have should be asked and answered. Our goal is not just a terrific orthodontic outcome ensuring a healthy, attractive smile, but also your anxiety-free comfort from start to finish.

4. **Finally, your treatment coordinator will explain the costs of the prescribed treatment program and discuss payment arrangements as needed**. Before proceeding, the next two appointments will be scheduled for the installation of braces and/or other treatment. As the saying goes, a journey of a thousand steps begins with the first one, and a task well begun is sooner done!

In total, you should allow about one hour for this entire initial consultation and exam.

If that seems like a lot, keep in mind there are *lifetime* health, appearance, and personality aspects of this. And it's not "installing tires"—not if it's done properly and expertly. Your son or daughter deserves a careful, thorough, and anxieties-eliminated experience. You want to make the best decisions for them.

Frankly, our practice and our process is not for everybody. We attract and "resonate with" parents who are quite serious about their responsibilities and committed to giving their child every possible advantage in life—certainly not unnecessary disadvantages. If you are that parent—and the fact that you took the trouble to obtain and read this book suggests it—then you are going to recognize that this is time well invested in the best possible results.

Call us at **804-704-8374** or go to **SmileRichmond.com** to schedule your own Customized White Orthodontics Smile Analysis.

"Andrew's older brothers (ages twenty-five and twenty-two) received orthodontic treatment from a different practice in the area and we wish we had discovered Dr. White's practice for them."

—MARY C.

Chapter Seven

Shouldn't There Be a Guarantee?

HEALTH CARE IS NOTORIOUS for no guarantees.

Surgeons have a dark-humor insiders' joke: dead patients can't sue.

If you've seen reality TV shows about plastic surgery, like the popular one airing as I wrote this, *Botched*, you know things can go horribly wrong.

Guarantees are controversial in all kinds of health care, including orthodontics. Many doctors are upset by the very idea. One huffed and puffed at me, "What do you think you're doing with this guarantee nonsense? We aren't operating a car shop, installing mufflers and guaranteeing them for five thousand miles. We are doctors, dammit."

His ego was mightily offended. But I doubt you will be, with the challenge of deciding who should be your family's *trusted* orthodontist. So, yes, I think there should be a guarantee! In fact, many guarantees!

1. **If you aren't satisfied with your son or daughter's orthodontic treatment, new smile outcome, or patient/parent experience, *our team of specialists will make it right, guaranteed.***

2. **Also, the quality of the orthodontic treatment itself is *guaranteed for life*.** If ever the proper teeth alignment originally achieved somehow begins to fail, we will welcome you back and do everything we can to correct the problem.

3. **You also have a safety in numbers guarantee.** The diagnostic and prescriptive methods and state-of-the-art technology and the braces products we use have been used by top orthodontists nationwide to treat over one million patients successfully.

4. **You also have my guarantee that *every* orthodontist and orthodontic assistant at my office has been not only academically educated but also *thoroughly* trained.** They all follow the same proven method to diagnose needs, plan the best and personalized treatments for every patient, and manage for best results from day one through after-care. There is nobody "learning on the job" with your child—ever. All patient care is supervised and reviewed by me. We also invest in frequent state-of-art clinical continuing education for our team exceeding all state licensing requirements. Above and beyond.

5. You also have *my guarantee of exceptional courtesy and customer service*. Yes, you are my patient, but

we can be honest about this—my practice is not just a health care provider, it is a *business*. As such, it has, in my opinion, one set of responsibilities to you as the parent of a patient and one set to the patient, including telling the whole truth and nothing but the truth, prescribing in the patient's best interest, and delivering the best possible treatment and outcomes. There's also a second, separate set of responsibilities to you as a customer, including access, convenience, responsiveness, and "red carpet service."

These five guarantees are included in your treatment program fee.

For starters, I can guarantee you the best, most thorough orthodontic exam, and I encourage coming in for it now.

Call us at **804-704-8374** or go to **SmileRichmond.com** to schedule your own Customized White Orthodontics Smile Analysis.

Chapter Eight

How to Get More Information

THERE ARE SEVERAL WAYS to get information about an orthodontic practice. First, I want to address the ways I don't recommend.

I don't recommend Yelp. Yelp is, unfortunately, not at all what it seems, and is frequently the subject of lawsuits from business owners, under regulatory scrutiny centered around the poorly policed manipulation of reviews, and has even been accused of the flooding of fake reviews—by "bots" no less! Some companies can use Yelp as competitive warfare while other companies turn around and sell the business owner under negative-review-assault "reputation management services." So, beware! Get the information you need from truly trusted sources.

Google can also be deceptive, though I admit it can be a valuable starting point. Rankings are manipulated by advertisements, websites, YouTube content, and what's called SEO, or search engine optimization. The only thing you know for sure about dentists or orthodontists who come up at the top in Google rankings in your community is that they are good at SEO or, more likely, good at paying somebody who is good at SEO. They're willing to spend money and willing to create a lot of content. Does that equate to certainty of the best diagnostic expertise, treatment, patient care, and customer service? Sometimes. Sometimes not.

So, first, the best thing to do is make certain you get all your questions answered by the orthodontist and the practice's treatment coordinator. Don't hold back. Put them on the spot. Be assertive. Don't feel you have to be deferential to the doctor! My own goal in this is to have every patient and every patient's parent *fully* knowledgeable about every aspect of the treatment so that they have *zero* anxiety.

Second, visit ExcellenceInOrthodontics.org. This is an organization of carefully chosen orthodontists joined together to provide carefully curated, vetted, authoritative, accurate, and understandable patient and parent information, hence its name. This can definitely help you decide on the questions you want answers to.

Finally, if you have a quick follow-up visit scheduled, these are wonderful opportunities to either ask questions you may have missed the first time, or to get further details from your orthodontist directly.

Now that we know where to get your most burning orthodontic questions answered, here are some simple tips I've amassed over the years to help you easily and effectively get the information you need:

How to Get Your Questions Answered

Make a list. The easiest way to get what you want is to know it in advance. Make a list of the various questions you have when they arise so you can quickly and easily go down the list to assure you've got the right answers for the right questions.

Bring it with you. Take the list with you when you go for your child's orthodontist visit. This way you have the questions at hand at the right place at the right time. If you're calling in to get answers, you can also have the list ready and tick off one question for every answer you receive.

Record the answers. If your orthodontist, or their receptionist, speaks too fast or you can't keep up while writing the answers down, why not record them? Your cell phone likely has a "record" feature, and if not, there are many affordable micro-recorders on the market today.

Double-check. Finally, make sure you have the right answer by double-checking with your orthodontist or their receptionist or assistant.

Knowing where to find the information you need is only half the battle; follow these tips and you'll know how to get what you're looking for as well.

Regardless of how many questions you have, or your comfort level with technology, phone calls, or in-person visits, your orthodontist should offer an option that fits your schedule and makes all your unresolved issues crystal clear.

Call us at **804-704-8374** or go to **SmileRichmond.com** to schedule your own Customized White Orthodontics Smile Analysis.

Chapter Nine

How to Pay For Orthodontic Treatment and Braces

YOU MAY HAVE NEVER needed braces. Or you may have needed them and gotten them. Or you may be among the tens of thousands of people in our generation who needed them but did not get them, perhaps because your family decided they couldn't afford them. Maybe they didn't consider it a priority and probably underestimated the lifelong results of the decision. You may not only have lived with a "hide your smile" habit unnecessarily, but you may have developed chronic jaw pain and headaches, difficulty chewing, or even periodontal disease that could have been prevented.

Regardless of which group you're in—and I hope it's not the third—I hope you will be making the best choices for your son or daughter today, without being hamstrung just by the finances. Truth is, parents pay out the same cost for a number of different things not nearly as vital as health or emotional well-being without blinking, mostly because it's paid in installments or just never really *considered*, like the monthly cost for minutes/data on mobile devices, added up for a year or two. The additional insurance cost and other costs when the teenager gets his driver's permit; after all, what's the choice? The cost of braces leaps up and stands there, all at one time. So, it can seem big. And it tempts thoughts of, "maybe later," or, "is this really necessary?"

I hope in the prior chapters I have succeeded at getting the "is it really necessary?" question erased. If there is visible need or if expert examination by an orthodontist and his explanation of what he finds can show you say it is advisable, it *is* necessary! It won't fix itself. It will probably get worse. It plagues a person's health, emotional well-being, social life, and career. It can link to very serious medical problems. *Necessary* is not really debatable.

Now let's tackle the ugly matter of the money.

I say "ugly" because nobody really likes talking about this. Most orthodontists are nervous about it. Parents are uncomfortable with it. If there is a financial obstacle to treatment, most people are reluctant to admit it, offer other excuses, and then can't be helped by the doctor. I think we have to trust each other. With me, this discussion is entirely confidential, in a "safe zone." Orthodontists are not Martians, by the way; *we* have kids, college tuitions that loom, and family budgets.

What Is a Reasonable Fee and Cost?

A complete treatment program, including braces, can cost anywhere from $4,000 to $10,000 or so. Most fall in between. Adjusted for inflation, these prices are actually *less than* braces decades ago, while the technology and quality has advanced. In costs it can prevent later, it's a bona fide bargain. TMJ treatments are expensive. Cosmetic dentistry work is expensive. Migraine headache drugs are expensive and have side effects.

For this investment, you will be getting the carefully selected, personalized solution to your child's irregularities and problems, prescribed using state-of-the-art digital technology along with the expertise of a specialist, and considerate, compassionate care from start to finish. Your investment includes a varying number of appointments plus the orthodontic appliance itself, after-care, and in my office, certain guarantees.

It's hard to really draw a fair comparison, but if you have any significant net worth, you can easily pay similar fees for the services of an attorney expert in estate planning. Most kitchen remodels cost considerably more. Where real expertise is involved and the stakes of getting it wrong are high, you can't escape professional level fees.

In this case, the $4,000 to $10,000 range is seen as perfectly reasonable by the overwhelming majority of parents that I talk to. Each year, we provide braces of one kind or another to countless patients. Even parents who shook their heads at the cost to start with tell me afterward that having witnessed everything we do to get the absolute best obtainable results, and seeing the outcome itself, they feel undercharged.

While it's never easy to part with such a sum, people do it every day for all sorts of less important things, like their new designer handbag, golf vacation, or suite of living room furniture. They'll pay for it outright or with their favorite credit card (getting the reward points in the bargain). If you put the orthodontic treatment program including braces on a typical credit card at the interest in play as I write this, and you choose to make only the minimum required monthly payment, your monthly payments will be relatively small.

Even tight budgets can accommodate this *when it is really important*. It's less than most families pay for their cable and streaming entertainment. For many, if they got all their Starbucks stops consolidated into one monthly bill, it would be more than this!

Health Spending Accounts (HSA) / Flex Spending Accounts (FSA)

The HSA allows you to set aside *pre-tax* dollars to be used for certain medical and health expenses for you or your family. They exist although restricted under the Affordable Care Act (Obamacare) as it stood in July of 2017. By the time you read this, the opportunity may have been expanded, as President Trump suggested. In any case, if you have accumulated money in an HSA, you can probably spend it on orthodontic treatment. If you don't have an HSA, you might want to start one. Information can be found online about existing or new accounts and their rules of use, at www.healthcare.gov.

Other kinds of FSAs are typically set up through your place of employment and similarly enable you to set aside pre-tax dollars for medical expenses. Sometimes, employers match contributions. Again, you can almost certainly tap funds from your FSA for your child's orthodontic care. Check with your employer about this.

If you have a tax accountant, you may want to consult with him about your HSA or FSA.

> **TIP**: How can you make the most out of your employer's flex-pay plan? First, make sure you understand how it works. Second, set aside flex-spending

dollars in advance of need, and if possible, make the maximum contributions. Many employers allow higher limits than you'd think without asking, as much as $2,500 to $5,000 per year. Be aware of "family status changes" allowed by your plan that may enable you to change the amount being moved pre-tax from your paychecks to your account anytime during the year rather than just once at the first of the year—so you could bump up the amount in months before the first orthodontic treatment. IMPORTANT: be aware of the balance and the loss of unused funds. In most cases, if you do not use these funds, you lose them, year to year. You usually have three months after the end of the calendar year to submit claims for eligible expenses from the previous year.

Insurance

These days, there are as many different types of insurance plans as there are patients in my office. I can't possibly speak to your unique and personal insurance policy without seeing it first but, in general, my experience tells me that "most" insurance policies cover "some" of your orthodontic expenses.

I realize that answer sounds very vague, but here are a couple of variables you need to answer before an insurance agent can help you determine what, how long, and how many procedures fall under your insurance:

- the type of procedure (braces, Invisalign, etc.)

- the duration of the procedure (two months, six months, a year, etc.)

- the cause of the procedure (a patient presenting with pain, a parent's concern, traumatic injury or accident, congenital birth defect like cleft lip or palate, etc.)

- the nature of the procedure (to correct pain/discomfort, cosmetic, etc.)

I can only partially answer this question, but talking to your insurance agent will help you get the right answers you need.

> **TIP**: Keep an insurance journal of every interaction with your carrier. Write down the date, time of call, name of the person you contacted, and the exact instructions or recommendations following the call. Later, if your insurance company doesn't remember what they told you, you'll have it accurately written down. If they still don't remember, ask them to pull the recorded audio tape from your previous call, so that you can accurately "remind" them of exactly what they told you.

Loans

If you qualify, we offer Care Credit, which can provide an unsecured, signature-only loan for the treatment program, with repayment over twelve to sixty months. You don't need to go anywhere else to apply or do paperwork; we can take care of it in my office.

If you have equity in your home, the lowest-cost loan option may be a home equity line of credit or second mortgage. See your own bank, or check out RocketMortgage at rocket.quickenloans. com. As of this writing, mortgage interest is at record lows.

Obviously, a private loan from a family member can be the easiest option. A lot of preteens' and teens' important orthodontic care is financed at the Bank of Grandma and Grandpa.

If the other options are difficult or unavailable, we will set up a weekly, bimonthly, or monthly "paycheck payment plan" with a comfortable monthly payment.

What If You Really, Really Can't Afford Braces?

I have compiled a list of eighteen ways you may be able to substantially reduce the cost of braces. Frankly, some of them are less than ideal, and most are not available through my office, but they could be helpful if your back is really up against a financial wall.

1. **Get braces in April or November and see if you can save a little extra by paying in full.** These are the months that orthodontists are the least busy, and it's when we have our most meetings (April–May). In November, everyone is getting ready for the holidays or the office is closed the week of Thanksgiving. By scheduling during the "off season," you can often find better deals with willing orthodontists.

2. **See if you can get a discount for not breaking any brackets.** Believe it or not, most orthodontists would

happily take $100 off your final bill if you don't break any appliances throughout treatment!

3. **New technology; better pricing.** See if you can be one of your orthodontist's first patients with a new technology and save some money on the lab fee or receive a discount for being a teaching case.

4. **See if your local dental school has an orthodontic program.** The treatment at such institutions is supervised by board-certified orthodontists (most of whom practice in the surrounding area). While you might spend a little more time in the chair as a teaching case, if you have the time, it might be well worth the wait because you can save up to *half the cost of traditional braces.*

5. **Ask your insurance plans when they send out their fee schedules to participating providers.** If the insurance company updates their fees or the orthodontist raises his or her fees to keep up with the cost of inflation, it might be around November in preparation for the next year.

6. **See your dentist every four to six months.** While you're wearing your braces, the extra cleaning each year can prevent tooth decay, a costly item to repair.

7. **Get your flex spending dollars in order with your employer.** If you set money aside in a flex plan, it may be "tax-free," but it comes with some stipulations: namely, you have to use it before the end of the year or else you lose it.

8. **See if you can get a second set of retainers from your orthodontist at the end of treatment.** Sometimes getting two sets of retainers at the same time can be cheaper than

buying a second set later in life when you lose or break your first set.

9. **See if your husband or wife has an insurance plan that covers braces.** Be sure to enroll in the plan with enough time to spare before your child needs braces, so that the procedure is not denied by your insurance company due to a waiting period.

10. **Ask for flexible financing options.** When you boil it down to the basics, your orthodontist really just wants to help you. Regardless of his specialty, your doctor spent way too much time in school *not* to love what he does. If you're easy to work with, keep your teeth clean, and avoid breaking your braces while you're wearing them, he or she will probably be thrilled to help you finance the care, or find another way to afford the investment.

11. **Do you have multiple kids in treatment?** If so, take advantage of that fact and see if you can get a family discount.

12. **If finances are extremely tight, you should check out the organizations that orthodontists have created to help provide pro-bono care, such as Smiles Change Lives.** There are even more foundations like this if you have a cleft palate or other facial anomalies, like the Rheam Foundation for Cleft and Craniofacial Research.

13. **School auctions, churches, or public service entities will often receive donations from local orthodontists wishing to donate a case to the school or organization for a fundraiser.** Checking around local school newsletters

or church bulletins for their upcoming silent auctions could be a great find! If you're unwilling to leave such things to chance, call your local schools or churches and ask them specifically if they have such a fund and, if so, how to apply/qualify.

14. **If you're thinking about a career change, apply at your local orthodontist's office.** Most orthodontists offer free braces to their staff and their children as an employee benefit! (And you never know, you could love your career *and* your child's new braces!)

15. **Military personnel, schoolteachers, and firefighters sometimes receive special courtesies in dental and orthodontic offices throughout the year.** Keep your ears open and you might save a few bucks or at least get a donation from the orthodontist to your organization.

16. **This tactic won't save you any money, but it could earn your organization or business some money if you have a newsletter, sports team, fund-raiser, or special event that needs a sponsor.** Ask your orthodontist. Most orthodontic offices are huge supporters of the communities in which they practice and would probably love to advertise with your organization.

17. **Got taxes?** Good! Why not use your tax refund to help pay for treatment in full and ask for a courtesy on the average fees associated with financing a full orthodontic case? In some areas, you can save as much as 10 percent on the cost of braces by simply saving your pennies and paying the entire bill at once, up front.

18. **Ask for more flexible financing through a third-party credit company like Chase Healthcare Advance, through CareCredit, or by using in-house financing through your orthodontist.** Most orthodontists will accept a reasonable down payment and split the remaining amount into easy monthly payments for your convenience. With automated withdrawals from a checking or savings account, you might be able to stretch the monthly payments out over a longer period to make each payment lower. Just don't be shocked if your orthodontist asks you to approve a credit check. A little homework up front can be well worth the effort when your monthly orthodontic bill is lower than your cell phone bill!

There's no doubt about it; braces can be expensive. However, now that you're armed with these eighteen massive, budget-saving tips, you won't need to decide between braces and your budget ever again!

Call us at **804-704-8374** or go to **SmileRichmond.com** to schedule your own Customized White Orthodontics Smile Analysis.

Chapter Ten

What Are the Treatment Options?

IF YOUR CHILD IS ready for orthodontic care, one of the first discussions to have with your orthodontist is which procedure is right for him or her; there might be more options than you had ever imagined.

If you're like most people, you associate orthodontists with braces, but these days, that is just one arm of what I or any orthodontist does. Here are some of the services most orthodontists will provide their patients with during the course of routine treatment:

- metal, tie-free braces

- lingual braces placed behind your teeth

- Invisalign clear removable aligners

- clear braces

- expanders to match jaw size and tooth size

- habit appliances to eliminate thumb sucking

- space maintainers

- retainers to prevent crowding and shifting of teeth

- headgear to help correct jaw alignment

- functional appliances to help improve facial balance

- early treatment and growth modification

- customized appliances designed uniquely for each patient

While many of these services may seem self-explanatory to you, several will probably not. In the following pages, I will try to elaborate on several of them, including:

- crossbite correction

- metal braces

- clear braces

- Invisalign

Crossbite Correction

As your child's teeth begin to grow in, there's a *lot* more at work than mere gum lines, tooth fairies, and molar size. How the jaw is shaped, when it develops, and even how "normally" it develops can all affect the placement and comfort of your child's teeth.

When the upper and lower teeth grow at different rates, or even when the lower jaw grows disproportionately with the upper jaw, something known as a "crossbite" can occur.

Your child might have a crossbite if, for instance, the lower jaw is out of line with the upper jaw (kind of like a box that won't close right because one of the hinges is bent).

Or perhaps on the right side of your child's mouth, the lower teeth "stick out" a little farther than the top teeth, making the upper teeth on that side overlap in turn.

Or maybe your child's upper and lower jaws are out of alignment so instead of the top and bottom front teeth meeting "naturally" as they should, the front teeth fall somewhat behind the lower teeth. This would be the reverse of an overbite.

As you might imagine, any or all of these developments can lead to short- and long-term discomfort for your child.

How, When, and Why Crossbites Form

You might be amazed to find out how many ways a crossbite can form as your child grows and develops during his or her formative years. Heredity is one key to jaw growth, or alignment, as is the size of your child's developing jaw.

Another factor that can contribute to the development of a potential crossbite is if it takes your child too long to lose his or her baby teeth. In some extreme cases, in fact, if it takes too long for your child to lose his baby teeth, another set of teeth can grow in behind them, throwing the alignment off and contributing to a crossbite.

Believe it or not, something as basic as whether your child breathes through her nose or her mouth can also contribute to a crossbite. While most children breathe through their noses, some children develop a habit early on of breathing through their mouths instead.

In children who breathe through their noses while they're sleeping, the tongue naturally rests on the roof of the mouth, promoting natural and proper upper jaw growth. When young children breathe through their mouths, however, the tongue relocates from the roof of the mouth to the bottom, removing that extra support and potentially contributing to reduced upper jaw bone growth; this can create the crossbite we spoke of previously.

How Can I Spot a Crossbite?

Although it sounds severe, and even painful from the description provide earlier, the effects of a crossbite can take time to manifest themselves. Still, here are some of the telltale signs your child might be cultivating, or already suffering from, a crossbite:

- snoring
- difficulty breathing
- chewing on one side of the mouth or the other
- signs of an underbite
- if your child's chin seems "off center" or disproportionate

How, When, and Why to Correct a Crossbite

Where should you start looking for treatment if you're concerned about your child's jaw development after reading this section? If you suspect your child might have a crossbite, approach your family dentist about a recommendation for a specialist such as an orthodontist.

There are many possible treatments available for a crossbite, and your orthodontist can work with you closely to make the right and specific decisions for you and your child.

When should you start? I believe you know my standard answer when it comes to questions like this one: *as early as possible*! The same way an auto mechanic would tell you to take care of that oil leak, bulging tire, or faulty timing belt sooner rather than later, myself and my colleagues in orthodontics will always favor early treatment to later.

Crossbites are often closely linked with other orthodontic issues, such as teeth alignment, jaw size, and growth, so naturally, the sooner you address any or all of these issues, the better.

Finally, why should you address a crossbite? Crossbites can lead to pain, discomfort, and a lack of confidence as your child begins to feel insecure or even ostracized because of this very treatable, very normal series of jaw and teeth developments.

Not only can crossbites become physically uncomfortable if left untreated, but if the misalignment or root cause of the bite isn't fixed early in childhood, then the child's appearance and, ultimately, confidence could be affected as the crossbite becomes more pronounced in adolescence.

Metal Braces

The fact is, metal braces still have a valued place in the orthodontic world, and despite advances and breakthroughs of products like Invisalign and even clear braces, they aren't going extinct anytime soon! This is because metal braces are very strong and can withstand most types of treatment. Today's metal braces are smaller, sleeker, and more polished than ever before.

"I have been so impressed with White Orthodontics. My daughter had a wonderful experience. The staff is very knowledgeable and extremely helpful. Dr. White has the best personality. I've recommended White Orthodontics to several people, and they have had the same experience. They are the very best in the Richmond area."

P. FISHER

Older, traditional metal braces require an elastic o-shaped rubber band, called a ligature, to hold the arch wire onto the bracket. These elastic ties collect more plaque and bacteria, making it harder for patients to clean the teeth and gums.

You may have heard of "speed braces." These are sometimes also referred to as "self-ligating brackets" or "tie-free braces." Self-ligating means that the brackets do not need the little o-shaped rubber bands (ligatures) or metal tie wires to hold the arch wire onto the bracket. Several companies have developed braces for holding the wires in place without ligatures.

By using self-ligation technology, the brackets allow the wire to slide back and forth. This advancement allows for fewer adjustments and fewer appointments. These types of braces do not need rubber bands to hold the arch wire in place. They use a "door" to secure the arch wire to the bracket. They're smaller than traditional metal and less food gets trapped around them when you eat.

Your orthodontist might use an advanced self-ligating bracket that does not require physical tightening of the wire to the braces. It's a twin bracket made of metal or clear ceramic and utilizes a special built-in clip. The pressure from specific types of arch wires activates the clip and delivers specific amounts of force to each tooth, resulting in fast, directed results.

Naturally, orthodontists are very excited about the hygiene benefits of these self-closing or tie-free metal braces. Patients are excited that their braces are small, smooth, and friction-free, and will straighten their teeth in fewer visits with less discomfort than braces with wires that are "tied-in."

Clear Braces

Ceramic braces are very strong and generally do not stain. Two popular brands are Clarity, made by 3M Unitek, and In-Ovation C, made by GAC. Adults like to choose ceramic because they "blend in" with the teeth and are less noticeable than metal. These are the type of braces actor Tom Cruise had.

Older types of ceramic braces required white or clear ligatures (tiny rubber bands) to hold the wire on to the braces. In-Ovation C is a revolutionary tie-free ceramic braces system that combines the same efficient tooth movement with exceptional aesthetics. Patients choosing In-Ovation C no longer have to decide between metal braces or clear braces that could stain.

Today's clear In-Ovation C braces are very aesthetic because they no longer require the small rubber bands that could stain with certain foods or drinks.

Adult Orthodontics

It's not uncommon for individuals who have undergone orthodontic treatment earlier in life to find their teeth have drifted out of alignment over the years. Most adults won't think twice about bleaching their teeth to roll back the effects of time. Yet few think about the role orthodontics can play.

Adults of all ages can enjoy the same cosmetic and health benefits of properly aligned teeth with appliances like the In-Ovation C system braces.

Improperly aligned teeth can do more than undermine your confidence. They can make proper cleaning and brushing more difficult, contribute to enamel loss, and even set the stage for more significant problems down the road. Fortunately, discrete treatment with In-Ovation C braces can help keep you aligned with a healthy, happy lifestyle.

The Solution Is Clear

Orthodontists believe every individual has the right to live their life with a smile they truly love, particularly children. Healthy, straight, and attractive smiles make your child happier and more self-confident. And isn't that what we all want for them?

In-Ovation C helps you achieve the smile of your dreams faster, easier, and more discretely than you ever imagined. Embrace the confidence that comes with beautifully aligned teeth and put your smile on display. Schedule a consultation and ask if In-Ovation C system braces are right for you.

The In-Ovation C system uses a free-sliding technology that places almost no pressure on your teeth as it gently corrects their alignment. Less pressure means a more comfortable treatment.

With In-Ovation C free-sliding braces, your treatment can proceed faster with fewer follow-up visits than traditional fixed wire braces.

Invisalign

Invisalign is a widely advertised, well-known, and popular braces product, and kids often know about it and ask parents and doctors for it by name. For many, it's as good an option as any other and sometimes even the best option.

Invisalign uses advanced, proprietary 3-D computer-imaging technology to "map" the entire span of treatment, from the present teeth alignment to the desired positioning, alignment, and smile. Clear aligners are custom made and based on the 3-D imaging. Invisalign has many features that have helped make it such a popular choice. The aligners are removable, even before a snack or meal as well as for general hygiene. There are no metal brackets or wires. Office visits for adjustments throughout the treatment program are fast, easy and painless. The thermoplastic aligners are virtually invisible. Over one million patients have been treated with Invisalign, and there is a special Invisalign system for teens.

Because Invisalign is computer mapped, there's sometimes the idea that anybody can install Invisalign and that all practitioners using Invisalign are the same. I have an important warning about this: during each stage of the complete treatment, only certain teeth are allowed to move. Which teeth move in what order, and the amount of time (days/weeks) needed for each successive set of aligners differs for each patient. *This* is what you rely on an expert orthodontist specializing in pediatric and juvenile care to decide. At the start, we determine whether your son or daughter is a good candidate for the Invisalign approach, or if they would be better served with different braces. You have to rely on *somebody* to tell you. I promise you, there are kids who've been hurried to Invisalign who were not good candidates for it.

Invisalign Teen

Much like the standard adult version, the Invisalign Teen System lets you do it the modern, hygienic way. Your new smile is created with the most innovative technology—a series of clear aligners that are custom-fit to your teeth.

The first thing you should know is that an average treatment takes about a year. Plus, your treatment can begin even if you don't have all of your permanent teeth. Invisalign Teen was designed to meet your needs.

Invisalign Teen aligners will snap on your child's teeth easily. They are comfortable and practically invisible. Invisalign Teen allows for permanent teeth to grow gently while continuously moving teeth in small increments. Aligners are worn for about two weeks and then swapped for a new pair.

Invisalign Teen aligners have a "Blue Dot Wear Indicator," designed to show an estimation of wear time. The dot is designed to fade until it's clear over a two-week period if you wear your aligners properly (meaning for twenty to twenty-two hours every day).

Invisalign Teen is designed to custom-fit to your child's teeth and go with his or her lifestyle. During your treatment, your child can keep smiling, playing sports, eating what he or she wants, and brushing and flossing normally because the aligners are removable. Plus, unlike traditional braces, the aligners are made of smooth plastic and move teeth gradually.

The aligners are replaceable if lost. That's right; you get up to six free individual aligners.

After your child's Invisalign Teen treatment, you may find his or her self-confidence boosted by their new smile and the change in their appearance. Some people even feel that way during the treatment. As you know, smiling has many benefits. It can help your child make a strong impression in lots of different social situations—at school, at work, or at a party.

Invisalign Teen really works. It helps correct a broad range of dental and orthodontic issues. You can get a confident smile without metal bands, brackets, or wires. It works on many kinds of conditions, including overly crowded or widely spaced teeth, crossbites, overbites, and underbites.

We've used Invisalign to successfully transform the smiles of many patients, but we do not prescribe it to everybody. After all, *popularity* should not govern medical care!

Trustworthy, Objective Advice

Our office is *not* "in the pocket of" or obligated to any of these providers of different braces products and technologies. We select and recommend what we believe is *the* most appropriate and beneficial choice for your child. We are happy to discuss the pros and cons of different ones, if your child has heart set on, say, Invisalign, because that's what a friend has, or based on information you've obtained.

Candidly, these manufacturers vary in price to the orthodontist (or dentist) based on volume purchase benchmarks, incentivizing concentration of as much use as possible to one product. Awards are given out to the highest volume buyers and users. It's borderline unseemly. It introduces temptation into the diagnostic and prescriptive process, and I never let us bow to such incentives and temptations. The number-one rule here is: what is absolutely best for the patient?

Call us at **804-704-8374** or go to **SmileRichmond.com** to schedule your own Customized White Orthodontics Smile Analysis.

"Dr. White and his team have been amazing.The genuine compassion and care we have received have made the experience as stress free as possible. We are thrilled with the results! We thank you for her new smile! What a huge difference—we couldn't have asked for better care."

J. NELMS

Chapter Eleven

How Difficult Is Living with Braces

REMEMBER, THIS ISN'T 1982. Or 1992. Today's braces aren't anything like yours if you had them decades ago. Today's orthodontic care is far more advanced, more sophisticated, and more patient-centered than any prior generation has experienced. If you had traditional metal braces twenty years or so ago, you experienced medieval torture. The dungeon is gone too, replaced by ultra-modern, comfortable, and patient-friendly offices. Out of the dark, into the light!

Living with braces is *not* going to be anywhere near as difficult as you might imagine.

Let's look at a few specific concerns.

Brushing and Hygiene

Modern braces, whether they're metal, flexible, or "invisible," are all actually made to fit the individual and facilitate easy, painless, thorough brushing. This means your child brushes pretty much the same as he would if he didn't have braces.

Here are some simple tips you can share with your child for the best results when brushing with braces on:

- Brush your teeth with a medium nylon toothbrush after you eat and before bed (no electric toothbrushes).[2]

- Brush, rinse, and look; if you find any areas that are not clean, brush them again.

- Brush your gums as you brush your teeth (massage and stimulate).

- Take extra care in the area between the gums and the braces because food caught and left there can cause swollen gums, cavities, discomfort, and permanent teeth stains.

- If no toothpaste is available, brush without.

- If you are unable to brush, rinse your mouth vigorously with water.

- Replace your old toothbrush when it gets worn out.

- It's absolutely essential you continue regular visits to your family dentist for checkups and cleanings throughout your orthodontic treatment!

---

2   At my office, you'll be provided with a home kit including the best toothbrush, toothpaste, and rinse.

Depending on the age of your child, you, the parent, may need to supervise the first few brushings with the braces in place. You should *not* have a whining, resistant, difficult child on your hands because of any of this. It should be painless, simple, and routine.

Forbidden Foods Your Child Must Avoid

After your child's orthodontic appliance/braces have been placed, the teeth are usually "tender" and sensitive for as few as three to as many as ten days: a *short* time. During these few days, softer foods are recommended: soups, macaroni, spaghetti, eggs, fish, Jell-O, yogurt. As needed, Tylenol or Advil are adequate in relieving any discomfort, taken an hour or so before eating.[3] Warm saltwater rinses can be helpful. We also provide a "soft white wax," a safe topical that eases gum discomfort.

For the entire duration of the braces being in place, I'd advise you to stay away from hard and sticky foods that can damage braces and may lengthen the time they have to be worn or even require extra office visits. Sugar-rich foods can make hygiene harder and cause calculus build-up and cavities. You're probably already monitoring and limiting your child's intake of such foods, so there's really nothing new under the sun here. But, for the record, here are the "featured items" that should be avoided during orthodontic treatment and wearing of braces:

---

3   Prescription pain pills with dangerous side effects are not needed. Any orthodontist or dentist easily prescribing such drugs is not to be trusted. As you are no doubt aware from the news, opioid addiction is rampant. Pain drugs are, contrary to early assertions by their manufacturers, proving to be extremely addictive for many people after nominal and legitimate use. I can't emphasize enough—we practice truly pain-free orthodontics.

1. **Rock-hard foods**: ice (don't chew ice!), nuts, popcorn (has hard kernels inside), peanut brittle, rock candy, whole apples and carrots (unless cut into bite sized pieces), corn on the cob, hard pretzels, hard rolls, hard taco shells.

2. **Extra-sticky foods**: Jolly Ranchers or Starbursts or similar candies, bubble gum, taffy, and sticky Cinnabon rolls.

3. **Very chewy foods**: pizza crust, beef jerky, gummy bears. Note: no chewing on pencils or pens.

4. **Super sugary foods and drinks**: soda pop with sugar, ice cream, most cookies, and cake. Yes, this is the worst of the forbidden foods. Some kids will give you a tough time. But there are sugar-free versions of all these kinds of foods, to be made, baked, or store-bought.

We will speak about this with your son or daughter and give them a printed list, but *you* will have to reinforce, monitor, and provide some substitute foods to prevent mutiny or months of sulking. Most kids get it, though. When they understand how short or long the number of weeks of wearing braces will turn out to be, how comfortable or uncomfortable wearing them is, how maintaining hygiene while wearing them is, and how their results are linked to them staying away from the short list of harmful foods, they are pretty responsible about it. Most parents who are initially really worried about this tell us later it wasn't the horror show they'd imagined.

Emergencies, Injuries, Travel, and Time Away from Home

Many "emergencies" actually aren't and can be easily and safely remedied at home. You are provided with a "What to Do in Case of the Five Common Emergencies" printed card, and you can always access the same information at our web site 24/7/365. You may also refer to the Orthodontic Treatment Reference Guide found on page 73 of my book, *When Will I Get My Braces Off?*

Common emergencies include the breaking of some part of the braces, eating something particularly damaging—even a McDonalds bun full of sesame seeds might feel like an emergency, or, early, a feeling of discomfort that worries something serious might be wrong. These are the sort of things addressed in the "What to Do" instructions.

If you do run up against an emergency that isn't easily managed with these instructions or if you can't wait for regular office hours, we have a special phone number to call that routes to a knowledgeable staff member directly and who will return your call within sixty minutes or less. All VIP Plan patients are guaranteed an office visit, if needed, same day, seven days a week. You are never left out to dry.

If your family or son or daughter are away from home and, say, they chomp down on a piece of toffee and break a piece of their braces, there is *always* a remedy. You are *not* going to cut your vacation short and rush to the airport! Again, often a remedy provided by our instructions can meet the urgent need until everybody gets back home. With some types of braces, we can FedEx temporary replacements. I also belong to a network of orthodontists with offices throughout the United States, which we can utilize in *the extremely rare instance* when getting to an orthodontist immediately is vital.

Here is just how good the appliances themselves and our management of orthodontic treatment has gotten. In 2016 to 2017:

- Ninety-eight percent of patients required *no* extra office visits for repairs, adjustments, care, or emergencies beyond their regularly scheduled office visits per their treatment plan.

- Eighty-five percent of patients called with questions, worries, or emergencies that were handled simply by advice and home remedy and/or waited without harm until the next regularly scheduled visit.

- Only 2 percent of patients had some problem or emergency requiring an extra, unscheduled office visit or express delivery of a temporary "patch" or solution to braces broken by sports, play, or other injury. We did FedEx a temporary braces repair part to a patient and his parents in South Africa while they were on a safari. I spent less than fifteen minutes on the phone with them when it arrived, and all was well!

Sports

Speaking of injuries, the question of sports versus braces worries kids and parents alike. These days, kids are *very* active in organized and school sports, some starting one as another's season is ending. You know this; you are coordinating the schedules and working as their unpaid chauffeur.

Good news: for every sport and every level of play, there is either an inexpensive off-the-shelf mouth guard or a slightly costlier, custom-fit mouth guard to provide an extra, suitable level of dental protection and to protect the braces themselves. In some sports, additional face masks or other equipment normally treated as an option can be added and used during the time period of the orthodontic treatment. Ask us for guidance for your child and their sport(s). Some mouth guards even come with insurance against dental injury, covering financial costs.

We have thought this through! For example, research reported in *Clinics in Sports Medicine*—from the Department of Neurology at Boston University School of Medicine—examined uses of different kinds of mouth guards and the rate of sports-related concussions. There was no significant difference in concussion risks found tied to different types of mouth guards. We can select the best one for your child, their sport, and the level of play and, if a factor, your budget with no worry about one choice instead of another affecting risk of concussion.

This, by the way, is typical of a good orthodontic specialist: attention to *every* detail. They should have a good knowledge of every ramification of wearing braces, clinical and technological advancements, and every patient or parent need. To be blunt, it's a practical impossibility for a general dentist to give the braces work he does on the side anywhere near this same level of all-in focus.

By the way, there are collegiate and pro athletes—even NFL players—getting orthodontic treatment and even wearing braces. If they can, your child can! You do *not* need the drama of stopping your child from playing the sports they're committed to because of their orthodontic treatment. Oh, and we even guarantee your office visits will not cause you to miss work or business responsibilities, nor cause your child to miss school or organized sports.

See, this *isn't* going to be difficult!

Tips for Helping Your Child Adjust to a Life with Braces

- **All the cool kids are doing it (or soon will be):** Braces are a very popular appliance during the middle school and high school years. Rather than focus on how he or she feels wearing braces, encourage your child to begin actively looking for other kids who are wearing braces. Chances are, they'll find lots more than they ever imagined!

- **Even famous people do it:** Gwen Stefani. Prince Harry. Drew Barrymore. Tom Cruise. Dakota Fanning. Danny Glover. The list of famous people who've worn braces—many of them as adults—could fill half this book. Share with your child how even the most famous people in the spotlight sometimes need a little help through braces.

- **Fast forward:** Many orthodontists provide a "before and after" consultant's session, much like a plastic surgeon. Digital pictures are often used to portray what the child's teeth might look like once the braces have been removed. Have your child focus on the "after" when he or she gets down about the "before" shots!

- **Be prepared:** Finally, create a "master list" of things your child likes to do, things that make them feel special, confident, brave, calm, relaxed, or excited. If you notice them feeling down, consult your list and make plans to do something special in the near future to boost their confidence level back to where you know it belongs!

Call us at **804-704-8374** or go to **SmileRichmond.com** to schedule your own Customized White Orthodontics Smile Analysis.

Chapter Twelve

Life After Braces: Retainers

SO, YOUR CHILD'S BRACES are off and they're ready to live a life full of confidence and good oral health. They may think, *I'm free! I'm free!* Well, not quite yet.

The selection of the right braces, the expert orthodontist, and the compliant wearing of the braces gets us about three-fourths of the way to where we want to be: a well-aligned, as-perfect-as-possible, healthy smile for life.

But after braces, there are retainers.

While many patients are understandably eager to be done with braces once they come off, the fact is, retainers do as much work—if not more—than the braces themselves. Straight teeth in proper alignment have to stay that way, and for that, retainers are a big help.

When the braces are removed, teeth can still shift if not helped through a period of adjustment to settle in. In fact, at White Orthodontics, we use a proprietary system similar to Invisalign we call "Clear Finish." This system involves a series of clear aligners to guide the teeth to their optimal and final positions. Then, retainers gently but purpose-fully remind the teeth to stay straight during this adjustment period. It's advised that nearly all patients who've gone through the time, work, and expense of braces will want to use fixed or removable retainers for months or years or even for life and continue to schedule regular orthodontic checkups. Some dentists doing braces won't tell you this, but I will. Years ago, clinicians believed that once teeth were straightened by braces, they would simply stay that way forever. New science says otherwise. In fact, teeth position shifting as we age is to be expected. Teeth naturally shift to the middle and crowd. So, retainers are actually extremely important in maintaining the new smile from braces. Any claims otherwise, by some "brand" of braces or any doctor, are flat-out false.

Retainers can play a role in:

- closing any gaps that may remain in the bite

- correcting any speech problems—sometimes occurring with a new bite or jaw position

- tongue thrust—where the tongue slips under the teeth while talking

- bruxism—grinding teeth while sleeping

As you can see, there's a lot more to this than just "installing and removing braces."

In post-braces monitoring and checkups, I tend to decide on the best kind of retainer for your child before the removal of the braces. Growth of the jaw following treatment (yes, the jaw is still growing in adolescents, to age eighteen or so), stabilization of the gums and bone tissues, pressures from lips and tongue, and other factors tell me what type of retainer should be worn and for how long. Retainers are made out of rubber, plastic, and sometimes, still, metal. They are custom made and fit as part of the complete orthodontic treatment. However, after the initial orthodontic exam, at the same time the best braces are being selected, it's usually possible, with a good degree of certainty, to predict the type of retainer(s) your child is going to need, and I'm happy to share that information with you at that time.

Some retainers are invisible or nearly invisible. There are clear plastic retainers. A *fixed* retainer is typically placed on the inside/back surfaces of the lower front teeth. At White Orthodontics, we are known for our custom-made, fixed retainers that fit snugly against the back of the lower front teeth. Since research clearly demonstrates that teeth crowd with age, we recommend the retainer be left in place indefinitely, or for as long as you want your teeth to remain straight. When your child hears "retainer" he will most likely picture a *removable* retainer. These make hygiene easy, are easily removed and cleaned daily, and can be removed for a sports activity. There are even "fashion retainers" now—popular with kids of different ages—in school colors, and some even with pictures on them! In my office, patients using different kinds of retainers also receive clear, flexible plastic retainers as a back up in case of damage to the main retainer or for occasional social functions where the preteen or teen "just can't be caught dead with a retainer in her mouth."

This is an important part of braces aftercare and part of the complete orthodontic treatment program personalized for your child.

Call us at **804-704-8374** or go to **SmileRichmond.com** to schedule your own Customized White Orthodontics Smile Analysis.

Chapter Thirteen

Let's Celebrate!

HAVING TO WEAR BRACES can last for six months to two years or more in certain cases. During the time your child has them, they may have moved from child to preteen or preteen to teen, at times feeling embarrassed by having them, and possibly missing out on some things. They probably gave up favorite foods and snacks. They at least had to be super-conscious of what they ate and didn't eat. It's been a long time since they could sink their teeth into an apple!

You endured whatever complaining there was. You traded time to the office visits. You dealt with the "uh-oh!" and the "now what did you do?" emergencies if there were any. And, of course, you paid the bill.

We like to see our patients celebrate getting their braces off. There are so many ways your child can celebrate, everything from writing a journal about their experience to recording a video that shares their experience and shows their new look.

Here are a few options your child may want to consider:

- **Throw a party**. Throwing a "braces are off" party is a great way to celebrate. They can invite their friends over, put out the foods that they've been longing for, and they can enjoy showing off those new straight teeth. Their friends will love being able to take part in the celebration.

- **Plan a photo shoot**. Your child deserves to show the world their new beautiful smile! Plan a photo shoot, so they can be one-on-one with a photographer and put their best smile forward. They'll get some great shots and can show all their friends on social media their new look.

- **Chew some gum**. Your child might have wanted to have gum for the longest time. Although it's not the best habit, they can take an afternoon to chew some gum and feel guilt and worry free. Chew to your heart's content!

- **Go caramel**. Now is the time your child can sink their teeth into something like a caramel apple. No more avoiding the caramel and cutting the apple into bite-sized pieces. Nope, they can actually eat a full caramel apple, right off the stick! They can get one at the mall or a carnival or even make one themselves. Either way, they'll love being able to bite into that sticky gooey sweetness worry free!

- **Picnic in the park**. Weather permitting, a picnic in the park will make for a fun celebration. Take some of your child's favorite outdoor games, invite the friends, and have a cooler filled with icy drinks. On the grill, you can plan for things like corn on the cob that your child had to largely avoid while wearing their braces. It will make for a memorable afternoon!

- **Have a potluck dinner**. Have your child's friends and family each bring a dish people with braces have to take precaution with. This will give them the chance to learn a little more about what you went through, and it'll be fun to see what options they come up with. Ask each of the guests to write down a comment about your child with or without her braces. Your potluck will be filled with interesting dishes, laughs, and a good time!

- **Relax**. What could be better than spending a couple of hours being pampered, or perhaps a round of golf or fishing out on the lake? Not much! Take your child out—celebrate them making it through their treatment. They'll walk out feeling and looking great!

Doing some of these things, such as chewing gum, may still not be good for your child's teeth or their body overall. But doing it on a special occasion, and not making a habit out of it, won't cause any harm.

Of course, nobody can celebrate unless we *started*. There really is no time like the present.

> Call us at **804-704-8374** or go to **SmileRichmond.com** to schedule your own Customized White Orthodontics Smile Analysis.

Chapter Fourteen

What About My Smile?

MOM, DAD, I'M NOT going to kid you: if braces and/or orthodontic treatment was advised when you were eight or ten or twelve and, for whatever reason, it didn't happen, and you now have misaligned teeth, periodontal problems because of them, a smile you often hide, and/or jaw/TMJ pain, it may *not* be an easy fix. It may *not* even be fixable with orthodontics or braces. But, often to the surprise of adults, braces—including invisible braces—can do a significant amount of good for people thirty, forty, or even fifty years old. You may still be able to go from an embarrassing smile you often hide to a beautiful smile you love! You'll also be able to enjoy better oral health, gently and gradually, over six to twelve months without having teeth pulled and without surgery. Many adults see ten years of age disappear from their faces!

The only way to know what the options are is with a complete, expert orthodontic exam.

While some offices may not actively seek adult patients, many will treat a lot of parents of patients, just like you, and a number of them come from referrals. You can arrange for your exam by speaking to any of the treatment coordinators at the office.

It's important to get your son or daughter the orthodontic care they need at the earliest time they are known to need it and for it to be the best care available. When that doesn't happen, it often comes around to really bite that person later in life!

Please don't ask them to hide their smile!

Call us at **804-704-8374** or go to **SmileRichmond.com** to schedule your own Customized White Orthodontics Smile Analysis.

"I can't say enough great things about White Orthodontics! Most importantly, they care about your child, who they are, and what they are interested in. The staff is patient beyond measure and willing to go the extra mile to make the process of wearing and maintaining braces as positive as possible!"

-M. BRADY

FAQ

Here is a handy resource guide of frequently asked questions and orthodontic terminology, many of which are answered throughout the book.

What might happen if your child's mouth doesn't quite "fit"?

The fact is, the sooner you straighten your child's smile, the faster it will develop as it should: straight, clean, and healthy!

Are there any celebrities who've worn braces?

Many! Gwen Stefani, Prince Harry, Drew Barrymore, Tom Cruise, Dakota Fanning, Danny Glover, and more.

Can I see what my child's straight teeth might look like before the procedure is done?

Yes! Digital pictures are often used to portray what the child's teeth might look like once the braces have been removed.

Will I be able to afford my child's braces?

Not only are most orthodontic procedures cheaper than ever, but insurance, payment plans, and a variety of other financing options make braces more affordable than they've ever been.

Will getting braces be painful for my child?

Not anymore! Modern technology—and choosing the right orthodontist—can ensure that your child enjoys a pain-free orthodontic experience.

How much school will my child miss because of braces?

Not much, actually. After initial visits and, barring the actual procedure itself, most visits and/or adjustments are routine and can take anywhere from fifteen to forty-five minutes.

Is it really such a big deal if my child has crooked teeth?

Unfortunately, yes. Eroding, crooked, or unaligned smiles can take time to happen, but the time to act is now. Orthodontic irregularities don't just heal on their own or "go away" if you ignore them.

What are some of the warning signs that my child might need to go to the orthodontist?

There are many, but here are a few of the most common: early or late loss of teeth, protruding teeth, grinding or clenching of teeth, and speech difficulty.

What kind of "side effects" are caused by crooked teeth?

Some of the more frequent ones I see include headaches, toothaches, mouth breathing, chipped or worn down teeth, snoring, and drooling.

What makes an orthodontist more qualified than a dentist?

Orthodontists are *dental specialists* who have completed two to three years of additional education beyond dental school to learn the proper way to align teeth and jaws.

Why should I choose a specialist for my child's orthodontic care?

Unique treatment requirements and otherwise difficult bite problems are common, everyday scenarios for your orthodontist. In the interest of receiving the most efficient and effective orthodontic treatment possible, choose an orthodontic specialist.

How do I know if my doctor is an orthodontist?

Only orthodontists can belong to the American Association of Orthodontists (AAO).

What is a treatment coordinator?

During your initial consultation(s), you will usually be assigned a patient contact person—we call this person a "treatment coordinator" in our office—with whom you will schedule appointments, confer with rescheduling, and of course, answer any and all questions you may have.

Why are follow-up visits important?

These are wonderful opportunities to either a) ask questions you may have missed the first time, or b) get further details from your orthodontist him- or herself.

Why is early treatment so important?

Age seven is the earliest time your orthodontist can determine future jaw and tooth alignment. That's because, at the age of seven, your child's upper and lower permanent front teeth are developing. These teeth set the stage for future jaw position and serious problems can develop if they come into the wrong position.

Is there such a thing as a child being too old for braces?

Actually, there is. Case in point: waiting to take your child to the orthodontist until they are twelve or thirteen can be very risky.

What if I don't believe in early orthodontics?

Well, you're entitled to your opinion, but this is like saying you don't believe in the sun. You can hide from it, pretend it's not there, or refuse to acknowledge it, but the simple fact remains. If you're not aware of the potential risks, you can get burnt.

Will my child actually need braces at seven?

Probably not. While I inform parents their child needs an initial exam at age seven, I also mention that most children *will not need braces until eleven to thirteen years of age.*

What is a crossbite?

When the upper and lower teeth grow at different rates, or even when the lower jaw grows disproportionately with the upper jaw, something known as a "crossbite" can occur.

Where should I start to look for treatment if I'm concerned about my child's jaw development?

If you suspect your child might have a crossbite or other issues, approach your family dentist and ask about orthodontics.

Why should I address a crossbite?

Crossbites can lead to pain, discomfort, and lack of confidence as your child begins to feel insecure or even ostracized because of this very treatable, very normal series of jaw and teeth developments.

What is Invisalign?

The Invisalign system is the virtually invisible way to straighten your teeth and achieve the dazzling smile you've always dreamed of. Using advanced 3-D computer-imaging technology, Invisalign depicts your complete treatment plan, from the initial position of your teeth to the final desired position.

What are the primary benefits of Invisalign?

Like the word that inspired them, Invisalign aligners are practically clear and as close to "invisible" as one can get. No one may even notice you're wearing these virtually invisible braces, making Invisalign a seamless fit with your lifestyle and day-to-day interactions with others.

How do I get started with Invisalign?

It's simple: just make an appointment with your local orthodontist for an initial consultation. Most doctors will offer a free initial consultation to see if you are a good candidate for Invisalign.

How will Invisalign effectively move my teeth?

Aligners are the foundation for, and work in unison with, the Invisalign system. Like brackets and arch wires are to braces, Invisalign aligners move teeth by using the appropriate placement of controlled force on your child's teeth.

How many patients are being treated with Invisalign?

More than one million patients worldwide have been treated with Invisalign. The number of Invisalign smiles grows daily.

Is Invisalign appropriate for my child?

Yes, especially because Invisalign now has a system designed specifically for teens!

How does Invisalign Teen work?

Aligners snap on your teeth easily. They are comfortable and practically invisible. Invisalign Teen allows permanent teeth to grow and gently and continuously moves your teeth in small increments. Aligners are worn for about two weeks, then you swap them for a new pair.

Why are metal braces still so popular?

Metal braces are very strong and can withstand most types of treatment. Today's metal braces are smaller, sleeker, and more polished than ever before.

Are so-called "clear braces" effective?

Ceramic braces are very strong and generally do not stain. Two popular brands are Clarity, made by 3M Unitek, and In-Ovation C, made by GAC. Adults like to choose ceramic braces because they "blend in" with the teeth and are less noticeable than metal. These are the types of braces actor Tom Cruise had.

Are clear braces appropriate for adults?

Absolutely! Adults of all ages can enjoy the same cosmetic and health benefits of properly aligned teeth with the In-Ovation C system and Clarity braces.

What are some of my payment options in addition to insurance?

One way many patients pay for their procedures is by utilizing the benefits of what is known as "flex spending," where their employer matches their spending commitment.

What if my child has a "braces emergency" before or after office hours?

If you are experiencing an orthodontic emergency that can't wait for regular office hours, most orthodontic offices have a special number to call, either before, during, or after business hours. If this information isn't given to you readily, ask how your doctor's office handles emergencies.

Can a salt water rinse help deal with irritation caused by braces?

Absolutely; warm saltwater rinses soothe the cheek lining, which can get aggravated by your child's braces.

How do I make a salt water rinse?

To make a salt water rinse, mix half a teaspoon of table salt in one cup of warm water. Stir until the salt is completely dissolved. Gently swish about a fourth of the cup in your mouth for thirty seconds. Make sure you force the water over the areas that feel sore. Then spit the water into the sink. Repeat until the entire cup is gone.

What if my child plays sports and needs a mouth guard?

The best advice for patients or parents looking for a mouth guard can be obtained from your pediatrician, dentist, pediatric dentist, orthodontist or oral surgeon. All of these specialists are uniquely trained to offer customized advice in order to help you prevent a sports-related dental or facial injury.

What about brushing with braces?

Here are some simple tips you can share with your child for the best results when brushing with braces on:

- Brush your teeth with a medium nylon toothbrush after you eat and before bed.

- Brush, rinse, and look; if you find any areas that are not clean, brush them again.

- Brush your gums as you brush your teeth (massage and stimulate).

- If no toothpaste is available, brush without.

- If you are unable to brush, rinse your mouth vigorously with water.

- Replace your old toothbrush when it gets worn out.

- It is absolutely essential that you continue regular visits to your family dentist for checkups and cleanings throughout your orthodontic treatment!

What type of foods should my child avoid while wearing braces?

There are four main types of food your child should avoid while wearing braces: (1) **hard foods**, like ice, popcorn, peanut brittle, rock candy, and corn on the cob, (2) **sticky foods**, like caramels, bubble gum, taffy, and suckers, (3) **chewy foods**, like pizza crust, crusty breads, beef jerky, and gummy bears, and (4) **sugary foods and drinks**, like cake, ice cream, cookies, pie, candy, and soda pop.

Why are retainers so important?

As we age, teeth naturally shift to the middle and crowd. Combined with late growth of the lower jaw, shifting of the teeth is expected following orthodontic treatment. Therefore, retainers are extremely important in the maintenance of your new smile following orthodontic treatment.

Resources

Before or after your consultation, you may want more information for yourself or your son or daughter. The following websites provide valuable insight to help you make the right decision for your child.

Braces.org is the "all about braces site" of the American Association of Orthodontists. This is the official regulatory body and professional association of orthodontists, and *only* orthodontists (*not* dentists) can be members. Here you will receive accurate, up-to-date information on orthodontics.

ExcellenceInOrthodontics.org is the elite association of orthodontists subscribing to a pledge of clinical and customer services excellence. A complete collection of information for patients and parents can be found here.

About the Author

DR. PAUL WHITE, DDS, was born and raised in Richmond, Virginia. As a second-generation dentist, Dr. White grew up working in his father's dental practice as a teenager, and worked his way through dental school providing dental hygiene services for other local dentists. After graduating from the Medical College of Virginia, Dr. White served in the U.S. Army Dental Corps, where he "defended the country against tooth decay," as he puts it.

When he returned to Richmond, Dr. White practiced general dentistry, and eventually developed a passion for understanding what made a healthy bite (occlusion). It was then that he decided to become an orthodontic specialist. He received training from Emory University in Atlanta, Georgia, and once again, returned to Richmond in 1992—this time, to establish his orthodontic practice: White Orthodontics.

Since then, Dr. White has been on a mission to dramatically improve the quality of orthodontic care in the Richmond area. He has continued to attend annual, post-graduate training and seminars, and is most proud of his training at the prestigious Roth-Williams Center for Functional Occlusion in San Francisco. It was there that Dr. White received highly special education and training in the diagnosis and treatment of TMJ dysfunction and bite disorders (malocclusions).

Throughout the years, Dr. White has developed a reputation for orthodontic excellence, and is the go-to specialist for patients in the Richmond area who suffer from TMJ dysfunction and headaches. Dr. White lectures extensively in Virginia and throughout the country, and is the author of the best-seller, *Beyond Straight Teeth*.

Dr. White has combined what he's learned from giants in the orthodontic field with the latest technologies to develop one of the most effective orthodontic systems in the country. He has successfully helped over ten thousand patients get the beautiful smile they want and, more importantly, the healthy bite they deserve.

THE
NEXT
STEP

Your Customized White Orthodontics Smile Analysis

When you are ready, I urge you to schedule your Customized Smile Analysis, complete with a complimentary consultation, safe, 3-D digital x-rays (a $249 value) an exam, and a report provided to you and your son or daughter—all without cost or obligation.

Call us at **804-704-8374** or go to **SmileRichmond.com**.

www.ingramcontent.com/pod-product-compliance
Lightning Source LLC
Jackson TN
JSHW011939131224
75386JS00041B/1461